Why Good Sex Matters

Why Good Sex Matters

......

Understanding the Neuroscience of Pleasure for a Smarter, Happier, and More Purpose-Filled Life

Nan Wise, PhD

Houghton Mifflin Harcourt
Boston   New York
2019

The information contained in this book is intended to provide helpful and informative material on the subject addressed. It is not intended to serve as a replacement for professional medical advice. Any use of the information in this book is at the reader's discretion. The author and publisher disclaim any and all liability arising directly and indirectly from the use or application of any information contained in this book.

For information about permission to reproduce selections from this book, write to trade.permissions@hmhco.com or to Permissions, Houghton Mifflin Harcourt Publishing Company, 3 Park Avenue, 19th Floor, New York, New York 10016.

hmhbooks.com

Library of Congress Cataloging-in-Publication Data
Names: Wise, Nan Ellen, author.
Title: Why good sex matters : understanding the neuroscience of pleasure for a smarter, happier, and more purpose-filled life / Nan Wise, PhD.
Description: Boston : Houghton Mifflin Harcourt, 2019. |
Includes bibliographical references and index.
Identifiers: LCCN 2019024930 (print) | LCCN 2019024931 (ebook) |
ISBN 9781328451309 (hardcover) | ISBN 9781328451316 (ebook)
Subjects: LCSH: Sex (Psychology) | Pleasure. | Sex (Biology) | Sex.
Classification: LCC BF692 .W535 2019 (print) | LCC BF692 (ebook) |
DDC 155.3/1 — dc23
LC record available at https://lccn.loc.gov/2019024930
LC ebook record available at https://lccn.loc.gov/2019024931

Book design by Chloe Foster

Printed in the United States of America
DOC 10 9 8 7 6 5 4 3 2 1

To my parents, Ruth and Norbert Jacobson.
Without you, there would be no us.

Contents

Introduction

W hy do you study sex?"

It's winter 2012. Having spent countless hours over the previous three years examining brain imaging studies that involve women donating their orgasms to science, including piloting my own study with endless hours in an fMRI machine, this isn't the first time I've heard this question. I have presented my pilot data to the Society for Neuroscience at their yearly gathering of twenty-thousand-plus brain nerds featuring a dozen or so special lectures given by the rock stars at the cutting edge of the hottest neuroscience topics. Although other neuroscientists have conducted studies on how the human brain responds to sexual arousal, only two labs have been crazy enough to go all the way and study the brain on the big "O." The media loved the results of my team's study, which showed that orgasm was associated with increased blood flow —and therefore more oxygen—to more than eighty regions of the brain. "Have an orgasm instead of doing a crossword," one outlet wrote, "It's better for your brain, says scientist." You would think that people would know more about the sexual brain in general and orgasm in particular by this point, but that is not the case.

The "female brain orgasm video," as it has come to be known, had so many hits it crashed the hosting website and went viral (you can Google it for a view). No doubt this video is what got the attention of the *Nightline* producers and why Juju Chang was now waiting outside my lab, ready to roll her cameras.

I am mildly agitated at the prospect of having to stop everything to make arrangements for the crew to witness one of our studies, but I am also eager to do the show because I believe we have an obligation to validate the importance of human sexuality — and this gives us the opportunity to show our work to a large national audience.

So, before we start up the fMRI, I think about how to respond to Juju's question, "Why do you study sex?"

This is the same question that I have been asked since I first got into the sex research biz. I've been asked this question in my own psychology department by colleagues who seem uncomfortable with our work and who have expressed the opinion that our participants must be "exhibitionists" — the same colleagues who on occasion let little comments, like "Hey, sex maniac," slip when they bump into me in the hall. It's the same question I am always answering to justify our work. But, in a way, this question is also my own — it's what has been nagging at my curiosity over the past thirty years, from when I first began working as a psychotherapist, then a sex therapist, and now as a neuroscientist. I've been investigating this question in all sorts of settings because it raises so many issues about happiness, health, well-being, and pleasure, and, yes, about sex itself. Indeed, that's why I am writing the book that you now hold in your hands.

The scan fortunately goes well in spite of all the distractions, yielding yet one more orgasm to add to my data. At the end of the clip, there I am in my lab coat, giving my final sound bite. "We live in a country where people are really obsessed about sex and also very hung up about it. I think we need to get over that!"

Juju seems to agree as her voice-over immediately chimes in, "Our sexual happiness, it seems, depends on it." So why do I study sex?

Sex is important for overall physical and emotional well-being. Yet we know less about human sexuality and the brain than we do about possible life in outer space. In fact, until we understand how sex is wired in the brain, we will not fully understand how genitals, especially female genitals, work, how to help people with sexual disorders, and how and why addiction and mood disorders take root.

Interestingly, this question never came up when I was a sex therapist working privately with women and men on their complications and challenges in the bedroom. Sure, I'd been interviewed by magazines and newspapers, and some of my more interesting cases as well as my approach to sex therapy have been featured in books. But no one ever seemed to ask me why I chose a career focused on sex in the first place. That all changed when I decided to go to graduate school and pursue a PhD in cognitive neuroscience with a focus on sex.

Why did I want to understand how the brain and sex relate? Really, it all started with a hunch that was formed during my clinical practice as a psychotherapist (this was before I specialized in sex therapy). The more I observed and tried to figure out the roots of unhappiness, dissatisfaction, and unease in the lives of my patients, the more I began to notice a common thread underlying the chief complaint that brought these patients to therapy. These people were all plagued to a greater or lesser degree with the inability to experience pleasure in life — a lack of enthusiasm, a deficit in well-being, and a decided inability to enjoy even the simple pleasures. *It was as if these people had lost their lust for life.* From a clinical perspective, they were in a state of anhedonia, the inability to experience pleasure and its satisfaction.

Year after year, throughout my practice, hundreds and hundreds of people have showed up in my office, trying to understand why they feel so flat, so angry, so irritable, so anxious, so depressed. Many reports in recent years both highlight and quantify an increase in anxiety, depression, suicide, and acts of violence. We see and hear these reports on the news, and many of us wonder if this is a blanket reaction to the ongoing drama surrounding the state of our country. But, as a clinician, I know that this rise in anxiety and psychological pain is both preexisting and progressing. Although most of us won't recognize it as anhedonia, this lack of interest and burned-out flatness of our emotions are part and parcel of the diminishment of satisfaction that underlies — and drives — more of the same. In other words, we can't solely blame what's going on in the world. In fact, it is highly probable that this epidemic of psychological pain and the associated overly triggered negative emotions have significantly contributed to the current political climate. When in an emotionally defensive state of mind, we don't make the best decisions. We feel desperate and fall into fear-driven, angry, and reactive behaviors. We get emotionally hijacked. We may even vote against our own interests. Yes — making decisions while caught up in a cascade of volatile emotions rarely presages reasoned, productive decision making, and we get caught in what can feel like a never-ending cycle.

Like the proverbial frog that doesn't notice that his warm bath is gradually heading toward the boiling point, we have become so habituated to anhedonia that we don't adequately recognize its presence. Then it just gets worse, stealing our propensity for joy, robbing us of sensual delight, blocking us from the release of sexual excitement. What used to give us pleasure now no longer carries enough friction to lift us out of the flatline state called emotional downregulation, when our biochemical systems have become imbalanced. The results? Anxiety, discomfort, withdrawal, and overreactions, to name a few. At a biological level, our nervous system has become so dysregulated that we literally can't feel pleasure and, in some cases, have even stopped seeking it.

When I would broach the subject of sexuality with my psychotherapy clients, most were deeply resistant to even addressing the very existence of their sexuality in the course of therapy. I always begin a new client relationship with the following questions: "How's your health? Your work? Your relationships? Your sex life?" This last question routinely seemed to elicit strong feelings of embarrassment, shame, and fear from my clients. And yet, I also found that when they started talking about their sexuality in sessions, we were able to get at the heart of their other issues more quickly and with more insight. Once this door opened, they wanted to know why they couldn't have satisfying sex, why they didn't even want sex, and what, if anything, they could do about it. If they were able to talk openly with me about sex, clients became empowered across the board to go deeper into revealing their authentic selves in the process. And, once this door was open, they became much more willing to open others.

Although some sexual issues have real physical causes, the root of what typically plagues clients can be traced to anhedonia. Like so much of our human experience, sex is biological, psychological, and social, and understanding the interplay of these three factors in our experience of sexual pleasure sheds important light on the role pleasure plays more broadly in our overall well-being. Indeed, I had a strong hunch that what I was observing in my clients and patients was what I was also beginning to see in both the neuroscience literature and in my own research. But first, I had to crack the code about anhedonia.

Our anhedonia can take many shapes. Never before have we been taking so many drugs — both prescription and substances of abuse — for what ails us. We are facing an unprecedented number of deaths as people attempt to self-medicate their psychological pain. We are also highly reactive, as evidenced by the recent rise in road rage, gun violence, domestic violence, sexual violence, and other outward signs of a culture going "postal." Indeed, over the past few years we've been reeling from one mass shooting after another, with scores of innocent people killed.

But most of us who experience anhedonia do so without this outward cry of rage and despair; indeed, the majority of people suffering from anhedonia do so in relative silence, living lives tangled up in a stew of negative emotions, unable to experience the pleasure that would break them free. Though this silent majority may be leading otherwise productive, successful lives, they also live with pain, sadness, worry, fear, and shame. And this emotional quicksand seems only to be getting worse — *fast*.

As Bob Dylan once said, you don't need a weatherman to know which way the wind blows. Just look around. Pain is everywhere: depression, anxiety, addiction, physical ailments, psychic strain, social isolation, financial stress, spiritual suffering. These negative emotions seem to be getting the best of us.

So how does this relate back to sex?

I began to notice that even when clients sought treatment of issues that were not related to sexuality, as I dug deeper, their sex lives were often impacted. And when people came in for treatment of sexual issues specifically, whether it be for the lack of sex altogether, low or no desire, or difficulty with erections or orgasm, something was out of whack with their emotions. Like clockwork, when someone's emotional life was askew, so too was their sex life, and when their emotional life was wonky, their sex life often suffered. Year after year, client after client, I observed that regardless of how high functioning a person might be in their life — in their career, for instance — if an emotional issue brought them into my office, there was also something wrong or missing in their sex lives and vice versa. I knew this connection between emotion and sex was no coincidence.

Indeed, I found my clients' sex lives to be an incredibly helpful touch-stone — whether they were seeking help for this issue or not — because sex, whether it's happening or not, is always so readily demonstrable and recognizable for people. A client may not realize that they are experiencing an emotional imbalance, but they do know if they can't orgasm. Our sex lives are often the bellwethers of our emotional issues.

I've always known instinctively that good sex is tied to happiness and well-being and bad sex or the absence of sex is a likely trigger of unhappiness, and this connection between good sex and happiness was showing up in my practice. The people who report having healthy or satisfying sex lives feel better, manifest less depression and anxiety, and experience an overall more complete sense of happiness in their lives.

It was this relationship between well-being and sex that proved to be one of the driving questions I wanted to investigate when I arrived at graduate school at fifty years old. I had a hunch that the brain is a big player in why sex makes us feel better or, to the contrary, why its absence makes us feel bad. I suspected that the key to studying this had to do with figuring out how the brain represents and processes pleasure. As I did a bit of digging, I discovered surprisingly little was known about how the brain responds to sexual pleasure. This gap in the scientific research fueled my fire. And I believed that although sex may not seem as important a topic as say cancer, AIDS, or dementia, studying sex from the vantage point of the brain had the potential to impact the everyday lives of many, many people and in ways that could be absolutely, positively life-altering.

Pursuing this giant hunch, I dived into a seven-year PhD program, spending copious hours doing lab research and using my free time to continue seeing clients. One of my first goals was to establish how sex —

good or bad — could be traced to activity in the brain. As I followed this thread, two distinct but inextricably linked ideas began to emerge: first, that the sexual issues that were so evident and pervasive in my clinical practice were tied to deep emotional or psychological unrest stemming from an imbalance in the core emotional systems of the brain; and second, that by examining the brain's activity during sex, I was beginning to get a fuller, more complete picture of how these imbalances in the brain in turn impact the body's experience of sex.

In the pages ahead, you are going to see just how pleasure and sex play out in the brain. You are going to see — just like I did in my lab — exactly how deep our pleasure pathway is tied to a set of deep core emotions that are wired into our brains. You will become familiar with how your brain operates — from its bottom, which works fast, almost automatically, to the midlevel, where we house our earliest learnings that show up in our behavior and attitudes toward pleasure and sex, to the top brain, our prefrontal cortex (PFC), which works more deliberately and slowly and tends to overthink, overworry, and overdo everything. Indeed, one of the most mind-blowing things you're going to learn is just how much we are still driven by this more primal emotional brain of ours — and it has a lot to do with why we are stuck in this state of anhedonia.

By looking through the lens of how our brains are wired for pleasure, we will learn how to reclaim our innate, biologically wired capacity and need for joy, fun, exuberance, curiosity, and humor in all aspects of our lives. Rediscovering this capacity for pleasure is key to fostering overall emotional and physical well-being. Are deeply pleasurable experiences important to you? Do you actively prioritize them? Do you cherish them when they strike? If not, you might well reconsider. Indeed, our relationship with our own sexuality can provide keen insight into how we think about pleasure, avoid pleasure, want pleasure, and resist pleasure. Since sex embodies pleasure, it affords us a particularly powerful lens through which to understand pleasure more broadly. It captures the complicated interplay between emotion, neural pathways, and personal experience — indeed all the factors that go into being able to have — and appreciate — true pleasure. And good sex, then, becomes the promise and the wonderful, delightful outcome!

By seeing all that's related to our sexual system you can retrace your path back to pleasure. This path also reveals outdated myths in how we define sexuality: it's not just for reproduction or for the purpose of relieving sexual tension. Our sexuality — like so many of our human processes and experiences — is deeply linked to our emotions, to our early experiences, to our current and past relationships. Because sex is biological, psychological, and social, it embodies so much of who we are and how we are doing at any given time.

Our relationship with our sexuality gives us a way to assess our capacity for pleasure, and, as we do so, evaluate the functioning of the emotional brain. I have come to see our sexual issues like the proverbial canary in the coal mine — an early warning sign of an emotional brain out of balance. Just as learning, memory, and decision making are all cognitive processes tied to emotional processes, our sexual experience — the drive for sex, the desire for sex, the avoidance of sex — are also tied to core emotional states that are wired into the brain. Uncovering these connections will not only show the way out of this pervasive state of anhedonia but will also show explicitly why sexual pleasure has the power and capacity to bring us a more complete happiness, one that is not just mindful but also full of all the sensations that the body brings to our experience.

Would you like to understand how to gain true satisfaction from both your daily experiences as well as sex itself? Would you like to understand how we are wired to need these pleasures in order to function at our best?

This book seeks to not only reveal the fundamental problem in how we think about sex and pleasure more broadly but also unlock the secrets about how women and men, regardless of age or orientation or inclination, arrived at this problematic relationship to their own experience of pleasure. The book begins by revealing how anhedonia shows up in the brain and how some of our lifestyle choices further undermine our capacity for all sorts of pleasure. You will see how the way that you think about and experience sex (or, alternatively, avoid it) reflects — and affects — the tonality and balance of your core emotions such as fear and anger, care and grief, lust and play, which are all part of our mammalian brains, driving the pleasure system. You will then gain a more accurate understanding of the inner workings of your sexual desire, emotional functioning, and capacity for pleasure. I've included many practical Good Sex Tools to help you resolve emotional issues related to pleasure and sex, connect with yourself and your partner so that you feel better, and learn how to question the limits that may be holding you back from fully experiencing your sexual potential. Some of these tools are exercises you do on your own; others you can do with your partner. All of them are designed to move you out of anhedonia and into pleasure.

Pleasure may sound complicated, but it isn't. We have a direct route to it through awareness of our core emotions. And our brain and its networks can be retrained and restored to once again reclaim pleasure, a state of mind attuned to satisfying sensations that allow you to actually like what you want and want what you like. As you map out your own path, you will learn the answers to questions like:

- What exactly is pleasure?
- What is the purpose of pleasure, in particular sexual pleasure?
- How is the brain wired for pleasure, pain, and other emotions?
- What is the link between pain and pleasure?

- How do our attitudes (both personal and societal) affect our experience of and capacity for sexual pleasure?
- How do our genes, environments, and nature/nurture interactions affect our capacity for sexual pleasure?
- How do the differences between men and women reinforce sexual misunderstandings?
- How can accessing our sexual potential make us smarter, happier, and more productive?
- How can a new understanding of sex lead to a more expanded way to experience pleasure in all aspects of our lives?

By exploring these questions, you will not only discover the healing power of healthy pleasures but also regain your lust for life. You will learn to unleash your own sexual potential and experience an ever-deepening, ever-expanding enjoyment of being an enlivened sexual being. Though we may seem to be in a pleasure crisis, when we follow our craving for pleasure, staying alert to all that it awakens in our bodies and brains, then we will no doubt discover a new frontier, one that I like to define as healthy hedonism, a place where pleasure is central and essential to all that we do in our lives.

Part One

......

The Pleasure Crisis and the Path to Healthy Hedonism

1

The Theft of Pleasure

Look anywhere in the media or on the streets of any major city, or suburb or small town for that matter, and we appear to be wholly focused on pleasure. Invitations to enjoy sex, food, sports, spas, exotic vacations, romantic escapes, and gamified apps abound, all promising a hit of relaxation, a high of excitement, an emotional or physical reprieve, and an answer to our aching need to destress. This environment encourages seeking pleasure in constant acquisitiveness — we're prompted to buy new clothes, tech toys, cars, or homes to an insatiable degree. Some reach for alcohol, drugs, or food for satisfaction. Others push their bodies to extremes, seeking pleasure in a new sport, workout, or diet.

Images both visual and textual are designed to direct our desire and our wallets to purchase pleasure. Some images, such as the more extreme example of online adult content and pornography, seem to provide a shortcut to pleasure. Television and online ads for pleasure-enabling medications pop up everywhere, reminding us that we can have pleasure when and wherever we want, regardless of our age or limitations on sexual function. Another version of this quick-fix mentality is the emergence of a seemingly endless parade of new dating apps that promise quick hookups, romance, and even wedded bliss at the touch of a finger.

From this vantage point, an anthropologist visiting our planet might conclude that ours is a culture gluttonous for pleasure and sexually ravenous. And yet, what I observe daily in my clinical practice is that for all of this pleasure-seeking behavior, all this *wanting* of pleasure, very few of us seem able to *fully experience* the sensations or satisfaction we seek.

Why, frustratingly, is this the case?

The Pleasure Shutdown

Given all the external stimuli found in our environments, it *seems* like we should be feeling tons of pleasure. But are we really that turned on? The answer, unfortunately, is no. In fact, our senses have become overwhelmed by this bombardment of easy-to-access, seemingly endless supply of quick-fix pleasures. Indeed, all of these promises of pleasure stand in direct contrast to the reality of our anhedonia.

Interspersed with these pleas or promises for pleasure is an equally consistent message: almost continual advertisements for antidepressant and antianxiety medications — not-so-subtle reminders that we are actually not well and need outside help because we are unhappy, anxious, stressed, and in pain — emotional, physical, and psychological.

I am certainly not alone in confronting this massive pain epidemic. It is evidenced directly in the enormous increase in the use of prescribed medications including antidepressants (up 400 percent since 1998) and opioid painkillers. Heroin and other illicit pleasure-seeking drugs have also undergone a dramatic increase in their intake — use that doubled between 2007 and 2012. A provisional report from the Centers for Disease Control in 2017 has indicated that the 70,237 overdose deaths reported in the US, many involving heroin, fentanyl, cocaine, metham-phetamine (up 22 percent from the previous year), and opioids (which have quadrupled since 1999), firmly establish overdoses as the leading cause of death among Americans below the age of fifty.

This epidemic impacted me personally when my thirty-nine-year-old nephew died of a fentanyl overdose. We had to wait for over five months just to get the official autopsy report because the medical examiner's office was so backed up with similar cases. A 2017 *New York Times* article reported that the chief forensic pathologist from New Hampshire, the state that had the most deaths per capita from synthetic opioids like fentanyl, has decided to leave his post to become an ordained deacon in reaction to the despair he faced daily on the job.

This drug use — both prescriptive and illegal — points to a similar root problem, though with different biologic causes. Numerous recent studies point to a worrying rise in the incidence of psychological pain. Indeed, one in five Americans will experience an episode of mental illness, while the rates of major depression and anxiety disorders steeply rise. And the clinical evidence in support of this rise crosses age groups, ethnic and racial groups, genders, and socioeconomic strata. These numbers and this growing reliance on medications to make us feel better all point in the same direction: a rise in *anhedonia*.

So, how did pleasure become so absent from our lives?

Our technologically driven, constantly connected culture reinforces this disruption of our pleasure system. Television binge-watching, non-stop texting, Snapchats, checking Instagram, and other repetitive behaviors that now happen almost automatically keep us distracted and numb, hijacking our neural pathways at critical points. In fact, "attention engineers" are being paid big money to keep us consuming the products tech culture sells by captivating us and keeping us clicking from site to site, app to app, sound bite to sound bite. Seduced into constantly seeking more, with little capacity to digest what we take in, we enter a state of "pleasure shutdown," never quite getting the opportunity to learn to feel our pleasures more fully, to savor the sensations — and to register whether this pleasure is indeed serving our well-being. Instead, we stay disconnected from our real needs and reach for quick pleasure fixes that only amp up our appetite to seek more, like being really hungry and getting quick whiffs of the smell of delicious foods without any sustenance. In always seeking, we also take away the opportunity to feel bad, uncomfortable, or truly needy — vital information that actually has a purpose: pain or discomfort is real information our brains need to register, process, and then fix.

This anhedonia, along with its accompanying anxiety and depression, disrupts the brain's ability to send and read these pain-pleasure signals, thereby disrupting whole networks reliant on their proper functioning.

As a therapist and clinical researcher, I witness this disruption on a daily basis. When I get up close to people and observe their *real* behavior and *real* emotional experience, I find that my patients not only cannot experience pleasure but they are often stuck in a cycle of pain — physical, psychological, spiritual, and psychic.

Simply put, the most basic, automatic enjoyments of life seem to be out of reach for millions of people. It is as if one of our most natural, necessary drives has become stunted, has dried up, has gone kaput. Yes — sex and other vehicles for pleasure are more available than they've ever been before, but few seem to reap their rewards. Instead, we see a population that is always seeking something just out of reach. With food, you may routinely eat long past when you feel full, but never really feel that you've enjoyed enough. When having sex, you may experience orgasm, but you never experience that intense, satisfying conclusion you recall from when you first fell in love. True pleasure — sexual or otherwise —

has become hard to find, and as a result, we have been cut off from an essential dimension of our capacity for happiness.

My Big Fat Panic Attack

In part, many of us have inherited a vulnerability to anhedonia, especially as it manifests as anxiety. In fact, the prominent American psychologist Dr. Martin Seligman has said that the predisposition to anxiety has been evolutionarily advantageous in that our ancestors who "worried" were more likely to live long enough to get their genes into the gene pool. Anxious preoccupations about having enough food and avoidance of predators kept them alive. But some of us who are "overly wired" to worry may have too much of a good thing — me included, as I come from a long line of anxious, anhedonic ancestors. In my immediate family, my sister has anxiety attacks and our mother has long suffered from them. It seems that my family's rite of passage to adulthood involves at least one major anxiety attack. My first panic attack occurred in the late fall of 1979, a few months after college graduation.

In retrospect that first panic attack was the result of a perfect storm. All of the necessary ingredients were present, including a medical issue that imbalanced my hormones (the biological), coupled with a time of developmental stress (graduation from college — one of the most difficult transitions young adults make), with a huge side order of trauma and loss. One of my best friends from college, who had managed to survive being shot in the head only two years earlier, had been killed in a freak accident on the New Jersey Turnpike while helping a motorist change a tire. My nervous system was primed to sizzle into a bona fide blowup.

At the time, I was taking graduate psychology courses as a nonmatriculating student while I figured out my career trajectory. During the summer, I had found an entry-level position as a mental health worker at a prestigious private psychiatric hospital. I was tasked with creating a "healing environment" by participating in groups and providing one-to-one supervision for the highest-risk patients. A few weeks before my attack, one of these patients, a young man just a few years older than me, escaped just after my shift and jumped off a bridge. I was devastated by his suicide. Haunted by a conversation with his parents during which I reassured them that their son was in good hands, I began ruminating on the tragedy. I thought I was okay, but I wasn't.

Nonetheless, I plowed forward. One evening, after downing multiple cups of coffee to keep myself alert, I headed off to campus to take an exam in neuropsychology. When I stopped into a Burger King to grab a meal, I was overcome with a sudden surge of panic. An impending sense of doom squeezed my chest along with a strong feeling of raw fear. I felt like I couldn't breathe, speak, or yell for help. I sat frozen, with my uneaten Whopper Jr. and Diet Coke in front of me, staring into space. Everyone and everything looked strangely terrifying, as if I were in a nightmare. The worst part, which I remember to this day, was the feeling of unreality. I didn't feel like I was in my own body. I was watching myself from afar, through a fog. When I gazed down at my own hands, they looked foreign, as if they didn't belong to me.

Later, I would realize that these experiences, known as depersonalization and assorted feelings of unreality, are common symptoms of intense anxiety. But back then, I thought I was losing my mind. I remember wondering whether I should drive back to the psych hospital and seek admission. I don't know how I managed to find my way to the car, and then to campus, steered by a sense of commitment on autopilot, and onto the exam (which I somehow aced).

When I went home that night, I was limp and devastated. My world had been inexorably changed, my sense of who I was damaged in a way I felt was irreparable. I didn't go to work for a few days, calling in sick. I wasn't sure I would be able to return to the job, even though prior to the panic attack I had been filled with enthusiasm and excitement about the opportunity.

The following week, back at work, I confided my panic attack to Ellen, a nurse on the admissions unit, who has since become a lifelong friend. When I said that I feared I was going crazy, she said, "Sorry, no easy outs for you. You're stuck with the rest of us. Welcome to the club." The club that Ellen referred to was for those who experience anxiety. Up until then, I'd had no idea how many others suffered similarly.

Subsequently, I've used that same line thousands of time when talking to clients. Panic attacks, which sometimes morph into the longer-term anxiety condition called generalized anxiety disorder (GAD for short), plague many otherwise healthy people. Although in some cases GAD can be truly disabling, I've learned how to keep it from stopping me in my tracks and undermining my confidence and motivation.

That first panic attack hurtled me into therapy. By the time I showed up in the office of a psychiatrist, I'd convinced myself that my symptoms were the harbinger of something dire, like schizophrenia. Halfway through that first meeting, the shrink smiled. "You've had a panic attack. That's all. And you also have first-year-medical-school syndrome."

I looked at him blankly. "But I'm not a medical student."

His smile widened. "But you're working with seriously ill patients, and you're new to this. You're doing what medical school students often do. They start thinking they have the symptoms they're studying. I don't know how I can convince you that you aren't crazy — but I'd bet my own medical license on it."

During the session, we identified some of the triggers precipitating the attack, including the recent death of my friend and the suicide at the hospital. Since I didn't seem to be suffering from something more serious and didn't need medication, he referred me to a psychotherapist.

My journey into psychotherapy has been both personal and professional. Over my now thirty-year career, this deep dive into the mind and the brain and my own anxiety, its roots and its behavioral sequelae, has landed me here, at a place where the underlying explanation of my own hair-trigger alarm system, as well as the inordinate amount of anhedonia in the world around me, has become startlingly clear. Which brings me back to why pleasure is so important — it's a necessary buffer to anxiety and stress and an antidote to anhedonia.

Anxiety, Pleasure, and Anhedonia in the Brain and Body

Indeed, when it comes to anxiety, there is definitely too much of a good thing. Persistent, unremitting anxiety will deplete your resources, both physical and emotional, until depression takes root and triggers or reinforces even more anhedonia. It's a vicious cycle of emotional dysregulation: the inability to have pleasure drains us of enthusiasm for life; anxiety and depression rob us of the appetite and enthusiasm to pursue pleasure; and these negative emotions keep feeding off of one another.

Clinically speaking, *anhedonia* is the inability to feel a satisfactory amount of pleasure in many if not most aspects of what would ordinarily be pleasurable in our lives, leaving people with a nebulous sense that something is just not right. In other words, neither our brain nor our body can experience the gratification of pleasurable sensations. Others may be able to feel some pleasurable sensation, but that feeling never registers sufficiently to provide satisfaction. Regardless of its manifestation, anhedonia points to a dysfunctional neural system that affects both the brain and the body. Indeed, I consider this vital, inseparable connection to be better captured as one's "brain-body," because they are so closely integrated.

When we untangle the neural web, parse out the blocks or triggers that cause the dysfunctional reactions (or lack of reactions), we gain insight into how the disruption of our pleasure system affects all dimensions of our lives: from the enjoyment of food, to the enjoyment of physical activities, to engagement in work and other intellectual or creative pursuits, the sense of wholeness that comes from real intimacy in our relationships. Think of anhedonia as a giant, numbing cloud pressing down from above, smothering your brain-body system so that it can't gather enough psychic energy to respond to sensual stimuli. You stay in emotional and physical lockdown, constrained and incapable of letting go into the pleasurable release of joy, camaraderie, excitement, curiosity, and adventure.

At a neurobiological level, people suffering from anhedonia and anxiety have lost the ability to regulate. Their biochemical systems no longer respond to natural modulators such as exercise, rewarding social interactions, sex, rest, meditation or other endorphin boosters that used to reset their biochemistry. So, when the natural remedies don't work, more and more people who want to feel good, less anxious, and more motivated in their daily lives turn to antidepressant and/or antianxiety medicines, which cannot address the related psychological and social issues. Though helpful at alleviating symptoms, the use of antidepressants surely masks the complexity of the pleasure problem.

Obviously, some medicines are necessary and lifesaving; they can mobilize the brain and help us climb out of a shutdown state. But just taking the medicine will not provide a complete solution to constant anxiety or anhedonia. We need to keep in mind that like pleasure, anhedonia is not just an emotional or mental construct; there's an underlying biological impact (a bit "chicken and the egg"). Essentially, people suffering from mild or extreme anhedonia have dysregulated chemical systems — including dysregulated dopamine and/or serotonin, dysfunction in opioid receptors, and high cortisol (if they are also experiencing anxiety).

In many ways, the brain-body is in a constant battle to stay in balance and regulate because of our ubiquitous experience of stress. On the one hand, short-term stressors are beneficial because they challenge us to adapt and encourage us to cope, grow, and become resilient. There is even a term for this — "eustress" — which literally means good stress. Short-term stress might include a work deadline, a child going through a tough time, a divorce, or a move. When we learn to tolerate such stress, we grow our resilience. However, when our brain-bodies begin to perceive all stress as equally threatening, these situational stressors can result in chronic "distress." When this happens, the brain-body responds with steady high cortisol (the stress hormone secreted by the adrenal glands), which further interferes with our capacity to relax and experience pleasure. Suffice it to say that many of us are having trouble experiencing pleasure because our biochemical systems have become overwhelmed by an out-of-whack stress response.

Each waking moment of our day asks our built-in stress response to adapt to the environment. Our brains release key brain chemicals called neurotransmitters — such as dopamine, norepinephrine, acetylcholine, glutamate, and GABA — to alter our biochemistries in either defense against stress or to optimize stress. When our stress responses become maladaptive, a cascade of negative effects occur, including anxiety, depression, energy depletion, sleep disruption, vulnerability to illnesses — both physical and mental (including addiction) — and can even hasten the process of aging.

Some people are particularly vulnerable to maladaptive stress responses, including those who are genetically prone to addiction. Born with highly reactive brain chemistry, they are especially sensitive to stress, and once they discover that substances dull the pain of stress, their seeking system interferes with their reward system. Unable to experience the natural "high" of positive feelings from a release of dopamine triggered by the experiences of everyday living, they come to rely on shortcuts: drugs or other addictive habits, which do not truly satisfy.

They get caught in a loop of seeking more and more and more, which often leads to escalating compulsive behaviors. Chinese Buddhists have described this situation as "chasing the hungry ghost," where tortured souls are stuck in a hell-like existence, driven by extreme emotion, unable to digest the nourishment (i.e., pleasurable release from pain) that they relentlessly seek.

In this way, addictive behaviors only drive yet more anhedonia — and even more compulsive behavior — reinforcing a cycle of misery. These people are in a constant seeking state — looking for an elusive, constantly higher pleasure "hit," which is no longer under their conscious control.

One of the reasons it's so difficult to "get out of" the anhedonia cycle is due to this complex interplay between the brain and the body. But, as we'll see, once aware, we can mobilize our top brain's capacities to consciously regulate our emotions that live in our brain's so-called basement and then reteach our midlevel new associations, behaviors, and habits. As a result, we will feel newly empowered. Ultimately, when we get our emotional system in check, we can lean on our top brain to help us reframe situations. Change can even be as simple as telling ourselves, "Go and meet your friends for coffee; that will make you feel better." This type of top-down command is one of the key ways to restore our pleasure system and get us on our way to healthy hedonism and elevate the importance of pleasure, sexual and otherwise.

What Is Pleasure, Anyway?

Historically, we've had a love-hate relationship with sex and pleasure — most likely rooted in the reality that sex and the resulting potential for procreation has been associated with grave danger for us Homo sapiens. The bigger cranial capacities (and larger-headed infants) that evolution endowed us with came with a high price — very high rates of maternal and infant death. This condition even has a name: the human obstetric dilemma. Even if a woman managed to survive giving birth to her big-headed offspring, childbed fever was a frequent complication that made childbearing so dangerous that preparation of a will was a common practice for the expectant mother. This danger is still buried in our evolutionary DNA and is rooted in our bodies. So how do we let go of that outdated association? By understanding pleasure for its own sake. If anhedonia is the absence of pleasure, hedonia is the embodiment of pleasure. Historically, the concept of hedonia has been described in relation to happiness. Aristotle defined pleasure using the Greek word hedonia to refer to the act of enjoyment and delight. The Greek word *hēdonē* also suggests pleasure and the absence of pain. The other dimension of happiness is what Aristotle termed eudaimonia, which, like its Greek root, emphasizes a life's purpose. From this point of view, then, happiness is achieved when a person has consciously developed a sense of meaning in his/her life and also experiences a sense of delight and enjoyment. In *The Nicomachean Ethics*, his classic book on the philosophy of ethics, Aristotle distinguishes between these two aspects of happiness, giving eudaimonia more meaning or virtue, and classifying hedonia, while acknowledging its important role in human experience, as less virtuous or valued.

Since that time, thinkers, psychologists, and other scientists have more or less kept this division between hedonia and eudaimonia as a way to discern between the overall types or sources of pleasure, but, to me, this distinction has only reinforced the binary view of pleasure itself: pleasure as associated with the body, as less than the mind or soul, as limited and less meaningful. Eudaimonia carries the heft, the virtue — its meaning is in and of itself attached to purpose — a "life well lived," it's been called. What this distinction actually misses is the important role that pleasures of mind and body play in our emotional lives — moving us toward what will be good for us and moving us away from painful or toxic experiences that will harm. Pleasure as an emotion is meant on some level to help us live more effectively.

We have many forms of pleasure that are stimulating and enjoyable. Is pleasure the sensual experience of the sun on your face or a breeze through an open window? Is it the enjoyment of eating a delicious meal? Is it the vigor of climbing a hill, running a marathon, or swimming across a pond? Is it the satisfaction that comes after completing an exam or a long, productive day at work? Is it the simple delight that comes from gazing at a transcendent piece of art or listening to a transportive piece of music? Is it the full physical release after passionate sex? Yes — these are all common or well-known *vehicles* that bring us pleasure. Indeed, how people experience pleasure takes as many forms as there are people in the world. The experience of pleasure can be described as sexual and sensual, intellectual and fanciful, physical and emotional. It is naturally subjective and can change over time.

From a neurobiological perspective, there are subjective and objective forms of pleasure in the brain. Primary pleasures are food, warmth, sex, safety. These are fundamental needs that we are hardwired to seek because they are about our survival. Their experience is sensory; it's stimulating; it arouses our bodies and brains. Animals experience these types of pleasures. "Higher-order" pleasures pull on more of our brain areas because these pleasures recruit motivation, learning, and reward pathways. Monetary, artistic, musical, altruistic, and transcendent pursuits or experiences give us pleasure because they are goal directed and meaningful to us. Animals don't experience these types of pleasures — they don't have an experience of the "self" or conscious awareness of self attributing meaning to these goals. These kinds of pleasures are also subjective and depend on our own subjective tastes and experiences.

The feeling of pleasure, however, is more internal, right? It can be a physical sensation but also a mental or emotional construct. With both our bodies and our brains we can discover, cultivate, and truly embrace all sorts of pleasure — including sex. Thankfully, without the threat of danger, sex can be something eminently good for us. And the more attuned we are, the more pleasure we will experience.

Our Ambivalence about Pleasure and How It Gets in Our Way

Our society has had a long, challenging relationship with pleasure. A recent study indicates that American adults are having sex less often than before, with an especially steep decline since the year 2000. This decline is significant even when you control for factors such as age, gender, and marital status. And to top it off, in spite of the media's portrayal of young people as freewheeling, casual sex-seeking, hookup artists, those born in the 1980s and 1990s are now the adults who are having less sex.

There is a clear paradox when it comes to our sexuality — a vexing approach/avoidance that I have come to characterize as a "lewd-prude" phenomenon. As much as we are reinforcing the need for mindful "sexual conduct," scores of people are coming forth to report sexual harassment and sexual abuse that has long been in the shadows. Sex has become for many a place of pain rather than pleasure. Unfortunately, as movements like #MeToo have uncovered, there is quite a long-standing disconnect between the code of behavior we preach and its effectiveness in our society, creating a kind of shadow culture where people act out negatively and harmfully around sex. And even those who have not had a traumatic sexual experience are impacted by this social component that reinforces a disconnect from pleasure.

Our culture has deep roots in a Calvinism that associates pleasure (especially sexual or sensual) with shame and places a higher value on stoicism. A number of recent studies have shown that modern-day

Americans, even those who aren't particularly religious, continue to be influenced by traditional Puritan-Protestant morality. This infuses us with a disdain for and discomfort with worldly sexual pleasures and an excess of pleasure in general. It is my experience that people are literally afraid to "indulge" in the release of pleasure — as they have been conditioned by culture or bad experiences to associate having pleasure with the threat of danger or punishment. It is as if having "too much fun" evokes the sense that feeling good is bad or shameful. This connection may be even more potent for women. Just a few generations ago, women who engaged in such behavior might have gotten burned at the stake. Confusingly, this attitude seems to be directly at odds with the commodification of sex that is equally ubiquitous in American culture; sex sells everything from books to booze to boob jobs, from Viagra to online porn to plastic surgery to rejuvenate our lady parts, from haute couture to celebrity-endorsed Kmart collections. Indeed, looking in a shopwindow, we might actually believe that this celebration of sexuality is the American way. But a gap certainly persists between this advertised celebration and what we personally associate with pleasure.

In distinguishing between happiness and pleasure, psychologist Dr. Margaret Paul, the creator of the Inner Bonding Program, makes a common and often misleading point about pleasure. She says,

> There is a huge difference between happiness and pleasure. Pleasure is a momentary feeling that comes from something external — a good meal, our stocks going up, making love and so on. Pleasure has to do with the positive experiences of our senses, and with good things happening. Pleasurable experiences can give us momentary feelings of happiness, but this happiness does not last long because it is dependent upon external events and experiences. We have to keep on having the good experiences — more food, more

drugs or alcohol, more money, more sex, more things — in order to feel pleasure. As a result, many people become addicted to these external experiences, needing more and more to feel a short-lived feeling of happiness.

This view of pleasure as being momentary and inconsequential is problematic and essentially inaccurate. It's deeply rooted in Western culture, stemming from religious thought extending back millennia, when pleasure was associated with sin, a life of intemperance, and the body being a source of evil or human weakness. Indeed, abstaining from sex was seen as a virtue. This binary view of body versus soul formed the underpinning of philosophical, religious, artistic, and even scientific thought for centuries. Alas, it lingers today.

But my bigger problem with this view of pleasure is that it implies that pleasure is optional and not as valuable, as say, happiness. From a neurobiological level, nothing could be farther from the truth. Pleasure is essential and critical to our emotional, physical, and mental well-being.

Our ambivalence about pleasure is most obvious in our conflict with sex. We are deeply into sex, but at the same time, deeply at odds with it, often misunderstanding our own urges, needs, and desires. We judge our sexual longings, we curtail our desires, and we cut ourselves off from all that it affords us. We convince ourselves that we just don't need it or want it. This is a problem that speaks to an unhappiness at our core and why redefining our relationship to sex and pleasure is so necessary.

Making Sex Important

Living without pleasure affects not only men and women in midlife and beyond, but also young men and women in their twenties, thirties, and forties, in the so-called prime of their lives.

Consider Matt, a young, handsome, and very sweet professional, who is constantly perusing dating apps in search of the "right" woman. He goes on a dozen new dates per month, and yet, his deep thirst for connection goes unquenched. Matt has sex with a lot of women but does so for a variety of reasons, including in part because he believes his dates expect him to, and he thus sometimes has trouble becoming aroused. (Counterintuitively, young men are among the biggest consumers of Viagra-type drugs.) These first dates often involve more than a few cocktails to loosen up, sometimes causing Matt to experience alcohol-induced performance issues and further complicating his view of these experiences.

Previously, a young man like this would be diagnosed as having intimacy or commitment issues, and to some extent, that may be true. But what looms larger is Matt's context: he is stuck in a cycle of *seeking* pleasure — romantic and sexual — without the understanding of how and why he can't actually *feel* the pleasure. The ferocious pace of modern dating — the condition of plenty that dating apps create — results in a situation where it's difficult to learn how to get to know each other, to build desire, to savor connection. It's a Catch-22: the pace of modern life makes it harder to slow down long enough to cultivate pleasure and savor its satisfaction.

Matt is in this exact position. His ability to be emotionally and physically intimate is being hijacked by an imbalance in his brain's basic emotional circuitry. What Matt doesn't know is that his frenetic *seeking* of connection is actually getting in the way of his *finding* it. On overdrive, all of his wanting has set off an alarm bell in the emotional basement of his brain, and when the alarm turns on, the sexual system shuts down, hence his erectile dysfunction.

The purpose of this seeking system that Matt is caught up in is to help us adapt, feel motivated, and be resilient. But if we don't know how to turn down the seeking and learn to like what we have, then we are forever looking and never enjoying what we have. Matt's anhedonic disruption shows up as a disconnection between too much seeking and very little satisfaction. Out of reach for him now are warm, fuzzy emotional connections that would help tamp down the seeking. Instead, he is stuck wanting and never gets the positive, fulfilling reward that would come from a real relationship, its intimacy, and the resulting calming and bonding experience that would in turn make him feel safe and secure enough to relax into spontaneous and juicy sexual functioning.

To resolve this situation, Matt has to uncover what is driving him to seek and never feel satisfied. The first step for him is to become aware of the emotional habits underlying the "speed dating" that keep him moving quickly from person to person, without time to get to know anyone in particular. As a hedge fund manager, everything in Matt's world moves quickly — an ongoing relentless influx of information about developments, national and global headlines to track, scores of emails to field, bets to make, probabilities to compute. Matt has become used to and then dependent on the fast-paced thrills and the buzz of taking risks and winning that go with his job.

But in his private life, the strategies that help him win in business bomb bigtime. He and his penis know on a deep level that no connections are being made; he also knows that he is stuck in a cycle. Fixated on the chase, he cannot shift and slow down long enough to think about choosing an appropriate partner who might actually make him happy. And his easy access to romantic or sexual connections is only reinforcing the hijacking of the brain networking that enables — and needs — a deeper or more drawn out path to pleasure.

Matt needs to break the cycle and get out of his anhedonic disruption by first becoming aware of how his bottom and midlevel minds are operating around these emotional and behavioral habits. Then he has to learn how to consciously enlist his top brain to change the frenetic pace of dating that's been preventing him from deepening his ability to be intimate with an appropriate partner. Once he becomes aware of the behavior patterns that have more or less been operating unconsciously, he is able to accept my coaching (more use of his top brain) and start to slow down and savor the opportunity to get to know each person without the pressure of rushing into sex. And once he eliminates the habit of racing into sexuality, he is able to let his heart and head discover who he feels not only attracted to, but comfortable with — and his sexuality will unfold seamlessly.

Disruptions in the brain basement, where the core emotions are generated, can impact sex in entirely other ways as well. Linda first came to see me because she had no desire for sex. She and her husband are in their early fifties. Their kids are grown and out of the house; they both enjoy satisfying careers — Linda works for a national charity organization and her husband, Phil, is an entertainment executive. This was supposed to be a time in their lives to reconnect, Linda tells me in frustration. When I ask her to describe how she feels about sex and about her husband, she seems a bit tongue-tied.

Finally, she says, "I don't understand what's going on with me. I want to want to have sex, but I just have no appetite. It's like the last thing on my mind. Phil and I used to hump like bunnies. But now, it's like I have fleeting moments when I feel the possibility of getting sexual, but when the time comes, the desire just disappears into thin air. I just seem to be pissed off and angry most of the time, like a low-level boil. Everything and anything gets me annoyed. Phil is a good guy overall, but we live like roommates. And I find I resent him a lot of the time. For dumb stuff. I end up feeling like a shrew. Not fun!"

I ask her what else she's angry about.

"I think I'm mad at myself, my body, how I didn't accomplish all that I wanted to — my friends tell me that it's not uncommon to lose your libido after menopause. I just don't think that's it."

Linda's on to something. Menopause can slow down some of the hormonal surges related to sex, but it does not have to wipe out sexual desire. In fact, for some women, menopause is a time of sexual renewal because there's more testosterone in ratio to the estrogen, which also explains why some women past menopause get more hairy and fiery.

After a couple of sessions, Linda and I begin to uncover more about her anger. Indeed, that's the thread that will ultimately lead to an explanation for her lack of desire: she's too angry for sex.

She feels depleted by years of taking care of others — raising kids while working, and now nursing aging parents. She's tired of focusing on others to the exclusion of herself. She is on the defensive and not at all in the mood to connect. This anger is great information in that it signals that it's time for a change. After years of not having her needs met, anger is what she turns to in order to avoid feeling needy and vulnerable. Menopause often comes along at a time when a woman is in flux in many ways — and when she needs to make big changes. So, while menopause is likely *not* the cause of Linda's anger or her lack of sexual desire, it makes sense that her frustration is coming to a proverbial head at this time in her life. But the big changes that Linda should be focusing on are to actually listen to the anger and trace it back to its roots. This intense emotion is a clue and will provide valuable information as she charts her way back to wanting sex and pleasure.

In short, Linda has to take off her anger goggles so that she can reframe how she thinks, sees, experiences people, and even reflects on her own memories. Up to this point, her anger has been skewing her perception of everything. And once upon a time, a bit of anger might have driven some of her sexual behavior; for instance, she does remember that early on in her marriage she and her husband used to fight and then have intense make-up sex. But that was years ago. Now Linda is burned out from perpetual anger and the stress that comes from years of poor self-care.

Her accumulated resentments have come to a low boil, and with that, her access to her playful sensuality and sexuality is blocked.

To get out of defense mode, Linda needs to feel safe, so that she can relax enough for her innate sexual desire to resurface. This starts with helping her learn how to safely unpack her anger. By acknowledging that she has a right to feel angry and that the anger has a positive function in getting her attention about what is out of balance, she can then be more mindful in paying attention to and tolerating the feelings without spilling into angry and distancing behaviors that sabotage her connections and joy. This is the first step of her healing process. Then, she will be able to feel relaxed and receptive to her innate desire to connect — sexually and otherwise.

Matt and Linda are not alone — many men and women find themselves in similar behavioral patterns, in which the core emotional issues fueling their anhedonia manifest in sexual problems. These core emotions include the powerful negative forces of fear, anger, and sadness — our defensive emotions that exist to signal threat and protect us from potential danger. But we have other core emotions that are just as potent — the affiliative emotions of connection, including lust, care, and play. Another primary emotional drive — called seeking — interacts with both the defensive and affiliative emotions and sends us out into the world to secure our basic needs. Together, these neural systems forge the basis for our emotional minds, as it were. And although we always know what is on our minds, we don't always know which mind we are in — are we stuck in the basement? Unaware of our midlevel mind's automatic behaviors? Or are we using our top brain to its full potential?

As we see with Matt, when the seeking system is overactive, he cannot enjoy what he's been seeking. And with Linda, when the defensive emotions like anger are running the show, we have little or no access to the affiliative systems that are our source of joy, fun, and connection — all of what make life pleasurable. Together, these core emotional drives play out in our daily lives, throughout our lives, and no more vividly than through sex.

My patients represent the vast majority of women and men who complain of inadequate sexual experiences, from loss of drive or desire to penises that don't work, an inability to orgasm or an orgasm that comes way too soon, pain with intercourse, or pain with the intimacy that comes along with sexual interactions. Estimates of how many individuals suffer from sexual problems vary widely, depending on how these "problems" are defined and how the information is collected, as well as a host of other variables. Suffice it to say, it is believed that sexual problems are among the most common psychological disorders affecting the general population. We've been told by sex experts that the cause of an inability to enjoy sex is sexual dysfunction, brought on by age, hormonal disruptions, or other diseases such as high blood pressure, diabetes, heart disease, or depression. And yes, these conditions all play a role in sexual shutdown. However, the underlying causes for sexual dysfunctions that impede desire and responsiveness can be traced to the brain and how the brain processes emotions. That's why sex is such a powerful way to untangle our mysterious relationship to pleasure, our complicated neural networks that make pain and pleasure interdependent, and the dance of powerful emotions that underlie all aspects of our lives.

To truly reclaim pleasure in our lives, especially in our sex lives, we need to understand how we are driven by the powerful emotions that operate in the brain.

2

The Sexual Route to Understanding Pleasure

The brain is not only the command center for sex, it's also a generator of pleasure. These two functions — enabling sex to happen and setting us up to actually experience pleasure from sex — are inextricably linked in both the brain and the body. This is why for the past twelve years I have been working in the lab to study what happens in the brain during sex.

Like many a scientist before me, I began my research by using myself as a guinea pig for my own studies. I had spent endless hours conducting brain-imaging studies of women having orgasms in the fMRI in order to understand more about how pleasure — in the ultimate form of an orgasm — plays out in the brain. The world-famous sex scientists Barry Komisaruk and Beverly Whipple collaborated on an initial study, and I joined the team to take the work forward.

My early results showed clearly that for all the involvement of the body in the production and experience of an orgasm, the brain was also having a very powerful experience. In fact, my research was showing that as genital stimulation led up to orgasm, numerous brain regions involved in processing sensations, emotions, rewards, and pleasure were becoming highly activated, with more and more brain areas lighting up, until at the apex of orgasm the brain looked like a Christmas tree. Capturing this evidence of blood flow to the brain also showed that an orgasm not only feels good but is good for us. We are meant to experience pleasure.

One of the original goals of my research was to fill a huge gap in the scientific literature — to figure out the basic sensory wiring of the female genitals. It's still hard for me to believe that this basic and important work was not done until 2011, when we published a study that systematically mapped the projections of the clitoris, anterior wall of the vagina, cervix, and nipple onto the somatosensory cortex (the area of the brain's cortex, in females and males, that is activated by any kind of touch). This is the same area of the brain that processes the input from parts of the body that are sensitive to temperature and pain. The somatosensory cortex is sometimes represented by a figure called the sensory homunculus, or "little man" — looking like a cartoonish Mick Jagger — all lips, fingers, and penis. Since the neurosurgeon Wilder Penfield originally mapped the somatosensory cortex in the 1950s, not much had been done to fine-tune the representation of genitals in the somatosensory cortex. And even less was known about what some have called the hermunculus, or "little woman," in the brain. And yet, this understudied area holds important clinical implications, not only for the treatment of pelvic pain disorders, sexual dysfunctions such as the inability to orgasm (anorgasmia), painful intercourse (dyspareunia), and low sexual desire (hypoactive sexual desire disorder), but also how these dysfunctions impact our overall well-being.

My research focused on what is happening in the brain during genital stimulation and orgasm, beginning with looking at orgasms from all sorts of angles: through clitoral self-stimulation, vaginal stimulation, cervical stimulation, and even orgasms through thought alone. Through my connections, I developed a unique pool of participants for our studies — women and men who experienced highly pleasurable and satisfying sex lives based on their sexual functioning and insight into their own pleasure systems. My "ladies and men of the lab" offered up their bodies and their brains in the service of scientific exploration.

My initial experiments clearly supported the notion that the "mind" is the most powerful sexual organ of all. When I had my participants simply *think* about stimulation of the genitals, the results indicated that they experienced subjective sexual arousal and their brains showed significant activation of the sensory and reward regions. Thinking about a speculum being inserted into the vagina doesn't do a thing for the brain at all, whereas imagining the insertion of a dildo lights up the brain just as if it was responding to actual pleasurable stimulation of the genitals!

The scans from the experiment showed activations of the paracentral lobule — where the sensations from the genitals are represented. They also showed major activation of the nucleus accumbens, which is ground zero of the brain's pleasure/reward system. Anything and everything that feels good activates this pleasure center, from food to sex to drugs to rock and roll. What this study showed was that it is possible to just think about sex and these brain areas become activated, ultimately confirming how powerful a sex organ the brain actually is.

While a handful of scientists have studied the brain during actual sexual behavior (most focusing on the arousal stage), my research established orgasm as a big brain event that interconnects disparate brain regions, including the complicated, multidimensional pleasure system.

My studies indicate the brain is so widely and strongly activated by orgasm, infusing nearly all regions with oxygen, that orgasm may serve as the best possible "exercise" for the brain. My research also suggests how the inability to experience this release robs us of a crucial way to destress and keep our bodies, emotions, and brains regulated and in sync. It may be just as important to our overall health to work out our sexual brains as it is to work out our physical bodies. The big takeaway? These studies give scientific support to the benefit of pleasure to our brains!

At the same time that orgasm is flooding your brain with oxygen — which is critical to healthy brain functioning — it is creating a cascade of nourishing neurotransmitters and neurohormones that bathe the nervous system with potently positive healing molecules. Your brain has its own internal feel-good system — endogenous (produced by your own brain) pain relievers and mood molecules that enhance your well-being and do good for your overall hormonal (endocrine) and physical functioning. These functions all point to why we have a wired-in pleasure system.

In these studies, I also wanted to understand more about female sexual response, which was so understudied, and how exactly the brain is involved. I looked at how some of my ladies of the lab responded under two different conditions: orgasm brought about when a woman stimulated her own genitals, and that induced by a partner's stimulation of her genitals. My results thus far indicate that there aren't any significant differences in the brain response based on how the orgasm was created. This finding was important because the only two labs in the world that studied orgasm had found very different results, most probably because of a variation in their experimental methods. Our first experiment used orgasms experienced through self stimulation. The other group using PET scans reported decreasing activity in certain (frontal) brain regions at orgasm through stimulation by a partner. My own dissertation work sought to solve this discrepancy in the literature by comparing orgasms elicited by both types of stimulation, those provided by the self and those provided by a partner; we found that our results showed that orgasms, no matter how elicited, consistently evoked tons of activity all over the brain, including the frontal regions. Specific neural networks are designed to generate orgasms and elicit pleasure and both are crucial to overall healthy function of our brain-bodies.

The Symbiosis of Pain and Pleasure

Much of our growing understanding of what enables pleasure — our drive for it and our ability to experience it and remember it — counter-intuitively comes from the more abundant research into pain. And when we look at this pleasure circuit more closely, we discover that the pathways for pleasure and pain are closely intertwined.

This interdependent relationship between pleasure and pain is part of our survival network: we are designed to feel both as a way to protect ourselves. Pleasure and pain, interconnected in the brain, function together as signals for us to pay attention and approach things that fulfill our needs and avoid that which poses harm. When these signals get disrupted or malfunction, we feel more vulnerable and anxious and not as confident in our ability to take care of ourselves — all symptoms of anhedonia. Feeling and registering pain and pleasure is critical in that it helps us stay grounded and in balance, both of which are necessary for the full experience of pleasure and the foundation of a life worth living.

While the pain system has its own dedicated transmitter, wired to pick up damage to the body, the sensory and emotional impulses that are sent and received overlap with those used to transmit pleasure. All young mammals have built-in pain pathways that are designed to both pick up on painful stimuli and also snuff it out with pleasure-enhancing chemicals. These built-in pain-inhibitory mechanisms stimulate brain regions that in turn release key internal opioid substances (endorphins and enkephalins) that make us feel good. So though pain functions as survival information, with its own direct line into the brain, signaling us to fight, flee, or freeze, pain-relief mechanisms that are inherently pleasurable are also wired in — to protect against this immobilization. In fact, the way our opioid system works showed up in my own research when genital stimulation and orgasm both stimulated the same regions. This observed activation of the pain-pleasure pathways provides clear evidence of the biological roots of the pain-relieving effects of genital stimulation. Indeed, this is one way our internal opioids help regulate pain in childbirth, when certain neurochemicals are released to buffer what might be even more painful. This tension between pain and pleasure is salient in the sexuality of people who enjoy forms of kink, including being spanked for pleasure. At a psychobiologic level, people who get satisfaction from pain tend to need more stimulation than others who might find intense stimulation too much — all of which point to the many gradations in the experience of sensation — what stimulates one person may be painful to another and vice versa.

Further exacerbating this connection between pain and pleasure is our difficulty with tolerating any measure of negative feelings. At the first sign of pain, we take an aspirin. At the first sign of emotional discomfort, we may be told to take an antidepressant. In fact, as a culture, we are encouraged to not feel too much of anything. In reality, this attitude about discomfort points to a profound misconception about how we experience pleasure.

When we avoid pain, we also learn to avoid pleasure, steering clear of sensual or sexual experiences that might elevate our desire. Instead, we go into our defenses, like Linda. Think of it this way: though they may lose a pet and mourn the loss, most people will eventually want to seek pleasure through another pet. For those people whose intolerance for pain is too much, they will avoid these feelings entirely by never seeking another pet. If you are trapped in a pleasure-seeking mode and you are desperately trying to avoid discomfort or emotional pain, the end result is that your experience of pleasure is even further diluted and numbed.

In other words, there is utility to both pain and pleasure — both are meant to keep our brain-bodies in homeostasis.

Our avoidance of feeling too much either pain or pleasure is strikingly obvious when clients first show up for therapy and seem disconnected from any kind of awareness of the sensations in their bodies. It is hard to get them to even respond to the simple question, "What are you noticing in your body as we discuss this issue?" Their blank stares in reaction to my query speak volumes. My life's work has taught me that the ability to notice, experience, and tolerate the sensations in the body that accompany the thoughts in the mind is critical to empowering wholeness and well-being. We dwell so much in our thoughts, our interpretations of our experiences, our strivings, and our expectations that we register very little of what is actually happening in the body. And when we do attend to our bodies, we often get caught up in the *wanting* (things to be different) instead of the *liking* (of how they are). When signals from the body are interrupted, the result is that there is no result. No response. No stirring of the imagination. No tingling. No desire. This is the state of anhedonia for many who have lost touch with the capacity for pleasure.

The Big Picture

Suffice it to say, we are just beginning to unravel the complicated nature of how the brain and body are connected during sex and also how our brains act as powerful mediators for our experience of pleasure. Although we know our brains are involved in and contribute to sex, my research suggests that our brains largely *control* sex and pleasure. As the evidence grows, the idea that the most important sex organ is the brain appears to be more accurate than we could have ever imagined. And the implications of the brain-body connection related to orgasm and sexual pleasure are simply enormous.

So, what does this research and discovery mean in the big picture? The brain does hold answers to our sexual problems and more than likely explains how we can refind our way back to pleasure — sexual and otherwise. Why? Sexual pleasure is the embodiment of an unconditioned response. We don't have to think about it; it is built into our brain-bodies so that we can instinctively seek sex. Just like how we don't need to learn to eat and drink; just like how we know inherently to fear and avoid pain, we are also wired to pursue sex. Sex is a pleasure that is necessary for the survival of the species. Although experience and learning leads to the unfolding of our sexuality over our lifespans and can help or hinder its expression, the ability to get pleasure from our genitals and to be sexual beings is part of the basic equipment that comes with being human.

What I began to realize as I delved more deeply into the neuroscience research was that we know very little about the basic emotional building blocks of our brains, particularly in regard to pleasure. Yet what I was seeing in the fMRI was leading me to hypothesize that by understanding how these systems play out in the brain and in the lives of people (namely my patients), I had a unique opportunity to understand how we are wired and how we could recapture our innate need and desire for pleasure. I surmised that the anhedonia was a result, in part, of imbalances in these core emotional systems. Trying to persuade ourselves through top-down techniques (which rely on the higher-order thinking skills of the top brain) cannot alone help us simply decide to relax and feel good. At this level, we all know what we should do: exercise more, lose weight, worry less, focus on the positive, change the self-defeating ways we think — the list goes on. But as much as we know what to do, all too often we aren't effective at harnessing our attention and our behaviors sufficiently to implement these changes. That's because we don't know how the basement of our brains, with out-of-balance emotional systems, infuse our thoughts, feelings, and drives in ways that self-defeat.

We need to enroll some other kind of brain resources to help regulate ourselves.

Helping people rebalance their out-of-whack wired-in emotional systems such that they can experience more satisfying pleasures in general, including good sex in particular, was the answer I saw time and again in my practice. Women and men who had arrived frustrated, depressed, and at their wit's end because of sexual desire or functioning issues were able to not only rediscover the tremendous joys of sexual pleasure but also get to the bottom of the underlying biologic, psychological, and relationship issues that had been in their way.

What Is Sex, Anyway?

Before going under the hood (i.e., inside the brain) to understand how sex and the pleasure circuit are being stymied, I think it's important that we get clear on what sex is. When I teach human sexuality courses to undergraduate and graduate students, I always begin by asking them a question: "So, what is sex?"

The look of the befuddlement on their faces is priceless. *Don't we all know what sex is?* The subsequent silence in the classroom speaks for itself.

My guess is that these students are more sex positive than typical folks but still need a safe container to speak about it openly. Before we unpack the definition of sex, I initiate a discussion about creating a safe, respectful environment for exploring the hot topics of sexuality (be it with undergraduates or graduate students in clinical sexology).

One brave soul usually speaks up first — most likely the kid minoring in LGBTQ studies. "Sex is intimacy between two people that usually culminates in some sort of involvement of the sex organs. Sex is when we have sex with other people. You know. Sex."

That's great, I say. What do you mean by "the sex organs"? Are you talking about the genitals? And does sex always involve some kind of contact with someone else's genitals?

Again, silence.

I push further. "What exactly does it mean to have sex with other people?"

The listing of sexual activities begins. Everyone agrees upfront that having intercourse is having *sex*. "So, getting laid is sex. What about oral sex? Is that sex?"

The class is divided. Some say yes, others disagree.

I then ask, "Those of you who don't think that oral sex is sex, would you be upset with your partner if he or she got some head from someone else?"

After a bit of squirming, everyone agrees that blowjobs or eating pussy probably involves sex.

"So, what about sexting?"

Again, the class is divided. And again, those who don't think of sexting as sex, when further queried, agree that they would be troubled should their significant other engage in sending or receiving sexy messages with anyone other than them.

Hmm. Interesting. My students seemed to be suggesting that sexting doesn't involve genitals in the sense of touching them nor involve any contact in the physical sense of the word. So, it is one thing when we talk about sex in general and another when we think about our level of comfort when our partners engage in activities that we don't particularly define as sexual. Clearly, how we define these terms is subjective.

So I follow up with another question: while we are on the topic of whether sex involves physical contact with someone else's genitals, do you think that that is always true? Does sex always involve some kind of contact with the genitals? Does it mean that there has to be some kind of friction?

They like that idea. One of the students suggests that that is a good operational definition of sex: genitals plus friction equals sex. "So, is making out sex? You know, the french kissing kind, with tongues and all?"

Again, the class is divided.

What about the partner test? "If your partner were making out with someone else, would it be cheating?"

Unanimous agreement: Kissing is cheating, especially the making out kind, which also implies that it is a form of sex.

Okay, so now we have established that sex needn't involve genitals — lips and tongues can suffice. So, sex has something to do with connection? Intimacy?

We start to unpack the notion that sex goes beyond the activities, the actual behaviors, and expands to involve some kind of connection between the people doing it. The emotional intimacy, closeness, the desire, the vulnerability, the fear, the awkwardness — these are all aspects of sexuality.

I continue. "So, sex has something to do with intimacy with other people? What about masturbation? Is that sex? It involves genital touching and friction. Is it sex, if you have it with yourself?"

One cool thing about masturbation, unlike sex with other people, is there is no problem with communication. We know what feels good. We know how to get the job done, at least in theory.

Nervous giggles.

There's more. Our feelings about masturbation may vary, but it's my experience that people need to learn how to play their own instruments before they can play in a band. This information is very important to discovering and laying down your own pleasure pathway.

We watch a trailer for a documentary called *A Sexplanation* in which the director, Alex Liu, who donated an orgasm to science in one of my studies, goes around the world talking about sex. It includes an interview with a gay Catholic priest living in Berkeley. The priest says that there is sex and then there is SEX.

SEX in capital letters is the stuff the students in the class apparently don't want their partners to do with other people; whereas sex, lowercase, as described by the priest, holds that we are all intrinsically sexual — that we are always connecting — always communing with others. The students seem to be getting the picture. Sex is bigger than genitals, bigger than friction. Sex is complicated. Sex means different things to different people. Being sexual comes along with being a human being. We are born already programmed to seek sexual connection. We are born with the capacity to find pleasure with and through our connection with our bodies and one another. Even babies in the womb touch their own genitals. Why? Because it feels good. Indeed, what feels good gets the attention of our brain.

We are intrinsically sexual beings.

Most people have experienced, while falling in love, this inherent part of our nature taking on a magnified role. Interactions with other people become infused with an unusual glow, whether it be with the charming barista at Starbucks or the sassy clerk at Costco or the handsome guy at the local dry cleaner. This feel-good glow is the kind of generalized and softer sexual energy that is potentially present in our everyday lives as alive, sexual beings. Sometimes we find that glow outside the chemistry of a new relationship, in moments when we feel deeply connected with someone who has listened to us deeply or revealed themselves in an unexpected, authentic moment. This is why some have called this kind of lowercase sex spiritual energy exchange — they think of it as a moment of blending boundaries and feeling connected with all of our clothes on.

But, even with all of these competing conceptions of sex, what's one of the most consistent features underlying our entire Q and A? Sex is always about pleasure — wanting it, seeking it, needing it, enjoying it. It's both physical and emotional. It happens in the body — and now we know, it also happens in the brain. In the pages ahead, we are going to look at how sex and pleasure both emerge from the brain first as emotions, and then ultimately, as experience felt through the body.

3

The Core Emotions in the Brain's Basement

At the most basic level, our brain can be divided between the bottom, which includes our limbic system, designed to automatically and without conscious thought defend us, protect us, and support our survival; the midlevel, where we store core emotional memories and conditioned responses that form basic learning and adaptations; and the top of the brain, with the PFC at its center, which is in charge of directing awareness, conscious thoughts and actions, and higher-order decision making around our behaviors.

My insight into the brain's processing systems originated in part from my specific work with an amazing neuroscientist, Jaak Panksepp. Panksepp's work is paradigm shifting due to his rigorous scientific exploration of the continuity of emotional wiring across animals and the way he relates this directly to core emotional circuits of the human brain. Even though Charles Darwin first blazed this trail in 1872 with *The Expression of the Emotions in Man and Animals,* in which he documented cross-species commonalities for the primary emotions of fear, anger, grief, joy,

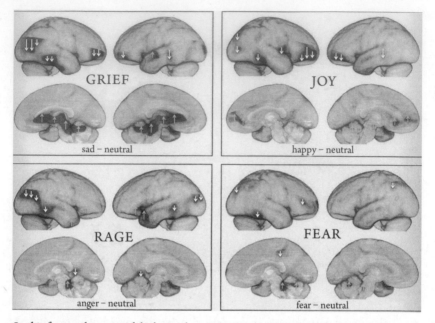

In this figure, the areas of the brain that are aroused or activated during the experience of the core emotional states of PANIC/GRIEF, JOY/PLAY, RAGE, and FEAR are indicated by arrows pointing up. The areas of the brain that are inhibited are indicated by arrows pointing down.

and play, the history of psychology is replete with resistance to the notion that animals could possibly experience emotion.

But Panksepp's work showed exactly this. He identified seven core emotions (or emotional systems) contained in "ancient subcortical" regions of the mammalian brain. He has shown through repeated studies that this hardwiring drives us to fulfill our needs and stay away from dangers. He established that all mammals have overlapping but distinct circuits buried in the deep, ancient parts of the brain — which, when experimentally stimulated (chemically or by weak electrical current), evoke specific emotions (responses that get us to move into the world) to meet our needs. These core emotional systems — SEEKING, FEAR, RAGE, PANIC/GRIEF, LUST, CARE, and PLAY — serve as the "primary colors" of our basic emotions, which, in concert with the higher

Basic Emotional Systems	Key Brain Areas	Key Neuromodulators
General Pos. Motivation SEEKING / Expectancy System	Nucleus Accumbens - VTA Mesolimbic and mesocortical outputs Lateral hypothalamus - PAG	DA (+), glutamate (+), opioids (+), neurotensin (+), orexin (+), Many other neuropeptides
RAGE / Anger	Medial amygdala to Bed Nucleus of Stria Terminalis (BNST). Medial and perifornical hypothalamic to PAG	Substance P (+), Ach (+), glutamate (+)
FEAR / Anxiety	Central & lateral amygdala to medial hypothalamus and dorsal PAG	Glutamate (+), DBI, CRF, CCK, alpha-MSH, NPY
LUST / Sexuality	Cortico-medial amygdala, BNST Preoptic hypothalamus, VMH, PAG	Sterolds (!), vasopressin, & oxytocin, LH-RH, CCK
CARE / Nurturance	Anterior cingulate, BNST Preoptic area, VTA, PAG	oxytocin (+), prolactin (+) dopamine (+), opioids (+/-)
PANIC / Separation	Anterior cingulate, BNST & preoptic area dorsomedial thalamus, PAG	opioids (-), oxytocin (-) prolactin (-), CRF (+) glutamate (+)
PLAY / Joy	Dorsomedial diencephalon parafascicular area, PAG	opioids (+/-), glutamate (+) Ach (+), cannabinoids, TRH?

This table shows where the seven core emotions are located in the brain and which neuromodulators (neurotransmitters and hormones) are associated with the respective core emotions.

brain regions, drive our emotional lives. (Panksepp always capitalizes these systems to bring attention to the discrete nature of their functioning and give them a concrete connotation.)

As you can see in the table above, these core emotional systems are not theoretical; indeed, Panksepp mapped them in the brain and also identified the neuromodulators that help them function.

Panksepp identifies three levels of emotional experience (he calls it the three-level mind). The first is made up of "primary process" psychological experiences that are the instinctual emotional responses that generate "raw" affects or core emotions built into our brains by evolution. Panksepp has shown that this "basement" level of emotional experience is evident in all other mammals (and some other vertebrates, too).

These "raw" emotions in the bottom of the brain are fast and are experienced vividly, by man or animal, even in instances where there is no capacity to "reflect" upon the emotions. All animals show fear, rage, attachment, and other emotional responses without the benefit of a souped-up neocortex, which permits higher-level reflections on the feelings. Even human babies born with a rare condition in which the neocortex does not develop exhibit these core emotions. These primary process emotions ensure our survival by motivating us to automatically seek to meet our basic physical needs for water, food, and air; sex and pleasure; safety and sleep. And these core emotional systems are directed to respond to sensory triggers for pleasurable or unpleasant feelings. If something is perceived as pleasant or pleasurable, our brain-body determines that it's safe or good for us. If it's deemed to be unpleasant or threatening, then our brain-body automatically avoids it. The perception of pleasure and pain are wired-in as automatic mechanisms. In other words, our higher brain does not have time to think through the satisfaction of these needs; they need to happen automatically. These raw feelings require no prior learning (neither animal nor human needs to be taught to fear or avoid pain or to seek and like pleasure). As Panksepp says, "pleasure and pain facilitate survival." And, as I have recently come to believe, pleasure facilitates our "thrival."

The next level of emotional experience, the "secondary processes," which I call the "midlevel," are built upon the foundation of the "raw" emotions and involve learning and memory processes. In contrast with our "core emotions," which are always experienced, the secondary processes largely occur nonconsciously. This is the territory of our behavioral and emotional habits, which are stubbornly affixed because, after repeated enactments, habits become almost automatic, below the hood of conscious awareness. This is also the territory of our "implicit" attitudes, which continue to drive our puritanical ambivalence about sexuality and pleasure.

And at the top of the brain is the slow, effortful processing Panksepp refers to as the "tertiary processes" that distinguish us from our non-human animal friends. As Panksepp was fond of saying, humans and animals are very similar at the bottom of the brain and very different at the top. The third level is where high-level cognitive processing occurs — and this is where we think we live. These top processes include our cognitive executive functions involving thoughts and planning (permitting us to reflect on what we have learned experientially); our ability to be aware of our experience (such that we can reflect on our emotions as opposed to simply experiencing them); our ability to choose our paths and intentions (in conjunction with working memory, which is essentially our conscious window on the world); and equip us with the potential to regulate our actions and behaviors. However, this high level of complex emotional experience is very much mediated by the other two, more basic levels. In other words, the brain's basement and midlevels must be working cooperatively for the higher-level functioning of the PFC to do its jobs well. This is what we mean by bottom-up learning. It starts from the senses up, is relatively automatic, and essentially drives our associations — pleasurable and painful — to the world around us.

Ideally, the top, mid, and bottom systems work together in a well-balanced network of communication and mutual support, with none being squashed or overly dominant. The top brain, with its conscious awareness and wisdom, guides and corrals the energy and stimulation of the core emotions in our bottom brain, while the midlevel continually creates stored patterns of behaviors — some of which may be getting in our way. So the core emotions are necessary to keep us current, informing us of our needs, motivating us to get out in the world, and driving us to stay in balance.

But anhedonia has created a cleft in this finely designed system. One way anhedonia disrupts the brain is by interfering with the core emotions that are generated in the bottom of the brain, especially those involving the limbic system's circuit of structures, including the hippocampus (which helps us remember important events); the amygdala (which tends to get excited when presented with strong emotional information, whether positive or negatively valenced); the hypothalamus (which among its many and important life-sustaining functions includes the production and regulation of the molecules that makes us exhilarated, furious, horny, or happy); and the cingulate gyrus (which majors in integrating sensory input involved in processing emotions and helping us to regulate our behaviors). Under chronic stress or anhedonia, the neural pathways involved become hypersensitive and take over, disabling the PFC's ability to calm itself down or otherwise regulate the intense emotions. In other cases, anhedonia overwhelms and dampens these core emotions, flattening them out — this is what happens when we walk around like heads on sticks or "flatline," unable to feel any kind of positive emotion. When this happens, it's as if the PFC has lost its ability to downregulate or send soothing signals from the bottom of the brain. We stay trapped in the bottom brain's activated emotional defensive systems, although we don't realize it. Our top brains become totally awash in the psychic pain of anhedonia.

When any one of the core emotional systems gets out of balance, the whole of our brain-body is affected. A helpful parallel to understanding how our emotional systems are functioning too well or not well enough is the immune system. A hyperfunctioning immune system can result in an autoimmune disease. An underfunctioning immune system leads to infection, disease, even cancer. Likewise, both overfunctioning and un-derfunctioning of these emotional systems can result in problems, includ-ing anxiety, depression, loss of motivation, and a stubborn lack of joy or happiness. When these systems are balanced, people feel flexible, nimble, and open to the enjoyments of life. Balanced emotional systems enable us to face calamities and even catastrophes with resilience, resourcefulness, and acceptance, ultimately empowering us to live more freely and fully.

When people become overwhelmed by their defenses, their emo-tional systems can end up shutting down — very much the same way that an animal freezes when there is no escape. It is the most evolution-arily primitive response of our oldest defenses. This is when people feel immobilized, may climb into bed in a state of depression, lose the ability to cope, and avoid anything and everything as a way of basic survival. On the other hand, depending on a person's individual wiring and circum-stances, the emotional systems can become overly reactive. This is when a person can explode such that rage takes over and shuts down the higher cortex. A minor example is an anger outburst. The extreme example is a crime of passion, when someone harms or kills a loved one. It can also fuel self-destructive behavior such as drug abuse or suicide attempts. I call this a limbic hijacking.

It was Panksepp's research into the significance of these core emotions that helped me bridge a gap in how I began to treat my own clients and understand how to turn the tide of anhedonia. Top-down talk therapy was only so helpful. The real solutions that began to appear in my prac-tice occurred when I began to show my patients how to pay attention to their own core emotional responses and integrate this information from the so-called top of their brains, their command centers. Not only did I see their anxiety, sadness, or depression begin to lift, but I also witnessed healing occur in their relationships and sex lives. When they learned to rebalance their bottom brain's core emotions with the top-down processes that typically want to take over, balance was restored, and anhedonia disappeared. They were once again able to feel the pleasures they sought.

Awareness of these three systems gives us a choice and an opportunity to observe and help regulate these core emotional needs. By recognizing that we have these core emotional systems at the bottom of our minds, we are better prepared to detect when they are driving us in ways that don't serve our well-being. This awareness also affords us another opportunity: to use the power of our conscious awareness and intelligence to harness the energy, vitality, and excitement of these seven core emotional systems. So, let's take a look at how these seven core emotions work.

Your Seven Emotional Systems

Understanding your seven core emotions is the first step to bringing your own brain-body into balance and returning to pleasure. The SEEKING system, which is the predominant system, manages and regulates the other systems. The other systems fall into two categories: the *defensive* emotions (FEAR, RAGE, PANIC/GRIEF), which protect our survival by cuing us in to potential threats or danger from outside ourselves; and the affiliative emotions (LUST, CARE, PLAY), which ensure our survival by driving us to connect through relationships with people (a reminder that we cannot survive alone). Together these seven core emotional states are wired into our human DNA.

#1 SEEKING

This system is what gives us enthusiasm and exuberance for life. It is what empowers us forward to explore and engage with the world in order to get all of our needs met. A clear demonstration of the potency of the SEEKING system has come from animal experimentation. When this system is artificially aroused through electrical or chemical stimulation, subjects will sustain repeated self-stimulation (sometimes at rates of one thousand times per hour, indicating that the animal "likes" the sensations elicited, but is ultimately not satisfied given the burst of repetitions it exhibits). They will also be triggered to seek pleasure in other ways.

In order to survive, we must automatically seek out what we need. This is true of food, air, water, safety, love, companionship, and sex. Because pleasure is embedded into these basic survival needs, the experience of SEEKING, under the right conditions, can be highly pleasurable. However, when we get stuck in the SEEKING system, we can start looking for the right things in all the wrong places!

In the brain, the SEEKING system acts like a motivation system, a network of signals communicating between the primary processes of the lower brain and the secondary processes of the midlevel brain (the parts of the brain involved in learning) to drive us to want what we need. Much of this wanting (neuroscientists call it "incentive salience") is very much tied to the brain's pleasure-reward system and the basic appetitive desires that reward us with pleasurable stimuli, reinforcing the motivation to keep wanting.

Of course, as humans, we can also be driven toward other, more emotionally complex and abstract pleasures as well — such as forming meaningful interpersonal relationships, defining ourselves through work or creative pursuits, and reaching for long-term goals that take planning and perseverance. Indeed, this kind of goal-directed behavior is what in part distinguishes us from other animals. However, as with all the core emotions, if the most basic wiring of our SEEKING system is disrupted, then no matter how much we aspire to lofty goals, we will still encounter problems with motivation, with attention, with enthusiasm and determination. Problems in the SEEKING system can take the form of procrastination, avoidance, endless daydreaming without actualizing. A disrupted SEEKING system can also look like an inability to take care of oneself, a drying up of appetite, and a turning away from the pleasures of sex.

In other words, when we have difficulty experiencing pleasure, there's always a disruption in the SEEKING system. And the converse is also true: when we have a properly functioning SEEKING system, our desire for pleasure and our motivation to seek pleasure — sexual and otherwise — jump-starts the entire system.

With anhedonia, there can be many triggers or causes for disruption of the SEEKING system, as this system also plays a role in negative emotions. It drives the motivation to get away from harm — flee when frightened — and mobilizes the ability to fight when presented with a situation in which we have to protect and defend ourselves or our young.

Driven by the neurotransmitter dopamine, our SEEKING system is meant to cue us to feel enthusiastic about going into the world to pursue what we need and want through experiences. When this system becomes overstimulated and hijacked by chronic stress and attention overload, a domino effect occurs, disrupting all the systems at once, making us hypervigilant, overly defensive, irritable, uneasy, and anxious.

#1 SEEKING

When this system is in balance, you will feel motivated, curious, and engaged in your relationships and pursuits. You are successfully able to access and activate your other emotional systems, both to fulfill needs and avoid perils in ways that are flexible and productive.

When it's underactive, you will experience lethargy, lack of motivation, procrastination, anhedonia, depression.

When it's overactive, you will have difficulty concentrating and will experience craving, dissatisfaction, and compulsive behaviors, which can lead to addiction.

....

#2 FEAR

We are born with an innate fear response designed to protect us from danger. As Panksepp points out, we do not need to learn to fear things; this response happens automatically. Researchers accidently stumbled upon the FEAR circuitry (without initially realizing it) while studying self-stimulation of the reward pathway. Animals whose FEAR circuits were electrically tweaked looked and acted in a manner that showed their absolute terror. When low-level electrical voltage was applied to their FEAR circuits, the animals exhibited freezing behavior; and with high-voltage application, the animals attempted to robustly and urgently flee (flight).

It makes sense that we come preloaded by nature with a robust danger/alarm system, otherwise our genes wouldn't have made it into the gene pool. All vertebrates have evolutionarily encoded the ability to recognize external threats that reliably cause pain or predict danger. For example, all animals (including us) are wired to fear pain. Pain, as Panksepp put it, universally provokes fear. But what constitutes other innate fears can be specific to the species. Rats and some other critters are hardwired to fear the smell of certain predators such as cats — even without previous exposure. The fear of predator odors helped animals avoid ending up as dinner at least some of the time. Rats are also wired to be afraid of loud noises and sudden movements.

As for people, babies — right out of the womb — become anxious when not securely held and will react negatively to loud noises. And as they mature a bit, they become afraid of being alone in the dark. Generally speaking for humans, our FEAR system is relatively flexible. Other than being innately afraid of pain, as well as some other evolutionarily based tendencies such as fear of heights, snakes, and spiders, we learn to fear other things through our experiences. But what is clear is that all mammals are exquisitely wired to quickly and robustly learn to respond to a vast array of stimuli that predict dangerous stuff — stuff we indeed come to FEAR.

The amygdala, a key player in fast, automatic emotional pathways, takes information from two places in the brain: directly from the sensory system via the thalamus, and from the cerebral cortex. Information from the thalamus reaches the amygdala quickly and acts as a rapid way to spark arousal in a scary situation. Information will also leave the thalamus to go to the visual and auditory cortices for processing and can also trigger emotion as a result of that processing. This second pathway is slower than the first. fMRI research has found the amygdala to be responsive to facial expressions of happiness, anger, and fear, but it is the most sensitive to fear. The amygdala seems to play a large role in becoming classically conditioned by fear (midlevel-brain learning!) of some situations or objects. This fear conditioning can be conscious or implicitly learned. And of course, there is always the possibility of using top-down cognitive abilities to harness or decrease fear when it is not warranted. Bear in mind that these top-down strategies, "literally thinking ourselves out of irrational fears," for example, are not always successful due to the potency of the emotions at the bottom of the brain.

Once conditioned, FEAR learning is set down in the midlevel mind (the systems involved in learning and forming memories); it is ferociously stubborn. Posttraumatic stress disorder (PTSD) is a good example of fear learning gone bad. Think of what used to be called "shell shock," the earliest label for this disorder. Soldiers came back from the World Wars with FEAR systems flexed one too many times, like a muscle that is overly trained. The consequences of being bombarded by direct threats of bodily harm and/or repeatedly witnessing horrendous images that sear the soul is an oversensitized alarm system. Take, for example, my own dad, who was a foot soldier in the trenches during World War Two. He saw some nasty stuff, very close up, like guys he had deeply bonded with get killed. When he first came home, every time a truck backfired, he hit the ground. Pure fear conditioning. Fortunately, this response gradually diminished over time. Dad dodged the PTSD bullet. But many aren't so lucky.

Not everyone so exposed goes on to develop full-blown PTSD, however. Like pretty much everything behavioral, there is an interaction between experience and genetic vulnerability. If you have sufficiently horrific experiences plus some kind of genetic wiring for the FEAR system that makes you overreactive, then you are likely to have lingering effects. In other words, the more sensitive your FEAR system, the more likely PTSD is to bloom.

And it doesn't take war, or a catastrophe like 9/11, or a natural disaster to cook up a bad case of PTSD. Trauma takes many forms. Children raised in toxic or unstable environments are vulnerable. Add to the mix repeated threats, emotional, sexual, or physical abuse, and you are looking at a kid primed for a very sensitive FEAR system.

The good news is that the comfort and stability that comes from our close, reliable relationships play an important role as buffers against fear. Yet people without this kind of emotional and social support may be in serious trouble. Persistent anxiety can take its toll on children's physical and emotional development, contributing to behavioral disorders, anxiety disorders, and predisposition to addictions as adults.

And recall for a moment, FEAR needn't be specific. Animals and humans can experience free-floating anxiety in the absence of an object to be feared. This is a basic inherent quality of our wiring. The symptoms of free-floating anxiety might not be as dramatic as PTSD or a panic attack, but free-floating anxiety is chronically stressful.

How does this stress response get so dysregulated and overreactive? When the brain-body picks up on some stimuli that triggers a stress response (i.e., fear), it begins to synthesize the available dopamine. Dopamine is then metabolically modified by various processes into what we typically think of as the stress hormones, epinephrine and norepinephrine (formerly known as adrenaline and noradrenaline, respectively). Then the adrenal glands release these two hormones, which initiate the classic "flight or fight" reaction. At the same time, cortisol, another hormone, is released by the pituitary gland. At first, cortisol helps to mobilize us: it alerts us to make a defensive move. But many of us may suffer from an overfunctioning of the FEAR system manifested as chronic stress.

....

#2 FEAR

When this system is in balance, you fear what you're supposed to fear and only to the extent warranted. For example, walking alone at night in a dark alley can be truly and appropriately scary, as is encountering a loud, angry dog. An upcoming work presentation, on the other hand, elicits some lesser but nonetheless motivating fear. Normal fear heightens our arousal system just enough to warn and mobilize us.

When it's overactive, your FEAR system is so tweaked that you may overreact to threats and end up depleted by chronic stress; this is common with generalized anxiety. Your exaggerated fear no longer serves you and becomes depleting and part of the problem.

When it's underactive, you will have difficulty handling threats appropriately and may, for instance, deny what is dangerous. You may also not be able to learn from negative feedback or punishment, which can be indicative of damage to the amygdala.

....

#3 RAGE

Of all the seven systems, RAGE is the most conceptually complex. It is decidedly the most challenging to study in both animals and people, albeit for different reasons. In animals, stimulating the RAGE circuits of the brain elicits fighting behaviors that could easily endanger the lives of the subjects. Rats will bite, and most animals will work to turn off stimulation of these circuits.

What makes RAGE hard to study in humans is the incredible complexity of what happens at the top of the brain that transforms, modifies, infuses, and alters the core, primary emotion wired in to the basement brain. Psychologists can't directly study the RAGE system in humans as it would require invasive brain surgery to directly stimulate the pathways that innervate the RAGE system, which would be highly unethical. There have been cases in which this circuitry has been accidentally stimulated in patients experiencing neurological disorders while having procedures done to determine functions of brain regions prior to neurosurgery, usually in cases of severe epilepsy or other pathology. What's been observed in these cases is that people experience electrical stimulation of these circuits as generally aversive — people will clench their jaws and report intense anger, while experiencing massive befuddlement, flooded with the raw affect of RAGE without any apparent reason.

But how do we cognitively experience RAGE and anger at the top of the brain — our conscious awareness? If you think about it, humans are meaning-making machines. We like to have a reason for why we do stuff or feel stuff, and in some instances, when lacking a sufficient explanation, we simply manufacture one. Think of the person who gets easily enraged when a car cuts in front of him; his brain quickly jumps to the conclusion that "he's an idiot, jerk, a-hole" — these perceptions are completely subjective and more than likely untrue. Based on this wiring, it must be a strange experience for the person whose RAGE circuitry is turned on electrically, apparently out of the blue.

Typically, we have to settle for indirect measures of RAGE such as self-reports of anger (potentially distorted by people's desire not to be seen as angry jerks), behavioral measures of "aggression" in the lab (very complicated for many reasons), or looking at aggressive behaviors as they spontaneously occur, after the fact, in society. With humans, experimental manipulations to induce significant rage or anger require deception and are therefore deemed potentially unethical. In hindsight, the now infamous Stanford prison experiment has shown to have caused long-term psychological damage.

RAGE is the raw substrate onto which anger, the more complex, cognitively infused emotion, is superimposed. RAGE circuits get turned on automatically — without learning — when an animal (or person) is pinned down, physically threatened, or their actions are restricted. Likewise, irritation to the surface of the body will elicit RAGE. So will blocking an animal or person's SEEKING behavior (i.e., taking away his or her freedom to do what she/he wants!). RAGE is also associated with being hungry, thirsty, or even horny — essentially when frustrated in the process of SEEKING. One way to conceptualize RAGE is as a reaction to being cornered, threatened, or constrained from getting access to important resources. We can become enRAGED when frustrated in pursuit of a prize or deprived of something juicy and rewarding that was expected. Children experience RAGE activation when a new sibling comes along and steals their thunder — the roots of sibling rivalry. We can become enRAGED when rejected by a loved one or ostracized by a social network. It is essentially a drive to get what is in the way, out of the way — frustration triggers RAGE.

RAGE does have positive functions — it's what can inspire outrage at unfairness, inequality, and mistreatment of our fellow human beings. Harnessed RAGE is a powerful deterrent and motivator. However, in our anhedonic culture, it often gets out of control, disrupting much more than we realize.

Anger, on the other hand, is way more nuanced and is infused with higher-level thoughts and beliefs, those we call "secondary processes," involving the midlevel mind's prior learning and experiences looming beneath and below the hood of awareness. Anger tends to be top heavy and influenced by thoughts, opinions, interpretations, judgments, and beliefs — feelings that nonhuman animals simply don't have the neural equipment to produce.

When these tertiary processes from higher brain sources are added to the mix, anger begins to sound something like "I am mad because" or "this shouldn't have happened because it's not fair." Like rage, we want to assign blame, which is why we tend to attribute significance to an object, person, or circumstance when we feel angry.

I've observed that many people don't feel entitled to feel angry unless they feel they have been wronged or victimized. One of the biggest challenges in relationship counseling is to teach people that they don't necessarily have to make a partner "wrong" to be angry at them since most of what we fight about isn't clearly an issue of right or wrong. Research has shown that most relationship disputes are over a difference of opinions, and of course, we tend to think our opinions are right!

Aggression is yet another story, with even more twists and turns. Picture a husband coming home unexpectedly from work to find his wife in bed with his best friend. He is so enraged that he lashes out and attacks the other man in the throes of a "limbic hijacking." This illustrates "angry aggression," where the drive is to hurt or destroy the source of his ire. A common factor of aggression is that we want to hurt, punish, retaliate, coerce, or control. Aside from "angry aggression," experts on the subject include fear aggression, maternal aggression (motivated by the need to protect one's young), irritable aggression (arising from persistent discomfort), sex-related aggression (motivated by jealousy or out-of-control lust), territorial aggression (protecting one's turf), and inter-male aggression (typically related to inter-male fighting over a female), which is usually centered on dominance. "Predatory" aggression, a form of aggression that shows up in animals, including people, when hunting for food, seems to be more of a function of the SEEKING system than the RAGE system. When hunting prey, an animal is not angry. It is focused on fulfilling the need to eat, and thus acts with aggression toward its source of food.

In humans, the various subtypes of aggression are built upon the roots of RAGE and then embellished well beyond the basics. Just watch the evening news to witness the full spectrum of how aggression is aggravated by competition for scarce resources, poverty, social injustice, and environmental stressors, all of which are further inflamed by different ideologies (at the top of the brain!). The way stories and information are reported in the media further sensitizes us to the dangers that loom and literally primes our defensive emotional systems (FEAR and RAGE) to be influenced more by feelings than facts. Sound familiar?

As we will examine more fully in chapter 8, there are real differences in the neural circuitry of male and female brains, resulting in differences in how our emotional systems engage. The short story here is that both males and females can be aggressive. Males tend to be both more assertive and more aggressive than females, in large part due to the effects of testosterone. Evidence for the role that testosterone plays in aggression comes from the results of infusing females with it. Women on "T" get just as assertive and aggressive as guys. We do know that males are more likely than females to become physically aggressive and perhaps even violent. On the other hand, females do their share of aggressive behavior, but it tends to be more subtle and in the realm of the interpersonal. Women appear to major in psychological pain, afflicted through ostracism or rejection of those deemed responsible for pissing them off.

#3 RAGE

When in balance, a RAGE system is associated with the ability to appropriately defend yourself against threats. It also allows you to take appropriate stands when angered that are constructive and facilitate resolution of conflicts.

When it's overactive, a RAGE system will cause a hair-trigger temper, elicit high hostility, and can also be linked to heart disease.

When it's underactive, a RAGE system suppresses your own defenses, allowing, for example, yourself to be bullied, or to not be able to stand up for yourself. An underactive RAGE system can present itself as a "victim" mentality.

#4 PANIC/GRIEF

Bruce Springsteen might be right—we are indeed "born to run." It seems we are also born to cry. Take any tiny animal (even a baby chick) away from its mother, and what you will evoke is heart-rending wails of separation distress, cries to be rescued, and desperate attempts to reunite with the absent parent (largely prompted by enrollment of the SEEK-ING system to search). Nature, in its infinite wisdom, knows that a defenseless newborn baby constitutes a tasty meal for a predator.

This system contributes to protecting our "life-sustaining social bonds" and is built into our brains to protect us by keeping us close to significant relationships and resources that are critical to physical survival and emotional "thrival." Built in to keep us connected to others —essential for a social animal—this is the system that gets triggered when we lose a loved one. It is the source of our grief and the neural substrate of heartbreak. For this reason, the PANIC/GRIEF system works alongside the CARE system: both are designed to ensure that we seek out companionship, care, and if we are lucky, community.

Early childhood experiences fundamentally shape the basic tonality of the PANIC/GRIEF system. While there may indeed be genetic predispositions that affect the reactivity of this system to begin with, the quality of our earliest social bonds with primary caretakers essentially forms the basis for how securely we view ourselves in the world, either dialing up the anxious style or dialing down the wired-in reactivity. Having our earliest needs met with attunement, warmth, and reliability, we grow into feeling that our needs are okay, and that people will be generally happy to help us get them met. Early caregiving that isn't so caring leaves lasting marks on this system such that the child is predisposed to insecurities and may cling in later years to loved ones, resulting in patterns that drive partners away, or even the avoidance altogether of deep sustaining relationships. Imbalances in this system often impact our "attachment styles." A secure or insecure attachment style predicts how confident we become in our capacity to get our needs met in the world, with and through our relationships with significant others, which in turn affects our overall tonality of PANIC/GRIEF and CARE.

....

#4 PANIC/GRIEF

When it's in balance, a PANIC/GRIEF system enables people to appropriately experience and tolerate the full range of their feelings, including the negative ones: sadness, disappointment, longing. Feeling all of our feelings is one of the surest signs of a high-functioning, resilient person.

When it's overactive, you might demonstrate an anxious attachment style, have difficulty separating from others, and in some cases, develop a panic disorder. An overactive PANIC/GRIEF system can be associated with trauma.

When it's underdeveloped, you might experience an inability to form and sustain close personal relationships and be avoidant or dismissive of people you know. This, as you will see, is also related to an inadequate or imbalanced CARE system.

....

#5 CARE

Bryan Ferry, the lead singer of the band Roxy Music, once sang, "Love is the drug and I need to score." Love is indeed a drug and we do need to score. We need to experience care (and love) in order to exist. As mammals, we also must invest a huge amount of time and energy in raising our offspring. And this doesn't apply just to mothers. Fathers of many species (including our own) are also equipped with the propensity to parent when dormant "maternal circuits" are activated by the addition of young into their nests. And it is the CARE system that shapes the development of altruism, compassion, and empathy — innate human capacities — in all of us.

The CARE system runs on internal opioids — our brains' own internally produced painkillers — the neurochemicals that are hardwired into our brains and bodies so that we attach to our young, our mates, our parents and friends. This is precisely the system that provides us with the natural feel-good chemicals that give us a sense of satisfaction and well-being. Panksepp has said that the physiology of motherhood is indeed the physiology of love. When we are anhedonic, we might be SEEKING a whole lot of stimulation — and craving a ton of stuff — but what we are really, truly hungry for is what we actually need. And what we actually need is what evolution has wired us for — social contact, connection, and love. Real face-to-face, eye-to-eye, flesh-to-flesh communion with our conspecifics (a fancy way of saying organisms of our own species). This urgent biological need is one that far too many are going without.

(In a pinch, connection with a dog or cat can be quite useful and deeply comforting. In fact, my own pup, Jilly, a skittish but very sweet Chihuahua, is a constant companion in my home and office, and instinctively sits on the laps of my clients as a therapy dog, making sessions even more soothing.)

When the CARE system becomes dysregulated, we feel emotional pain, lack a feeling of well-being, and become detached from others — even those we *think* we love and care about. We are vulnerable to addiction (essentially the conditioned learning of bad habits) when our internal opioid system is not functioning properly (and some people seem to be genetically wired with inherited deficiencies in the CARE systems). That results in reliance on external drugs (or compulsive sex or eating or something else) to ease the pain. With anhedonia, our CARE systems are compromised. We either withdraw from our important relationships or sabotage them, isolating ourselves further. Too little care prevents us from experiencing enjoyment with another person; too much care blocks our libido and stifles our ability to experience spontaneous play and enjoyment. Too much care for others can also undermine healthy self-care. Bringing this system into balance is crucial for good sex, as it is for the invitation of pleasure.

....

#5 CARE

When your CARE system is in balance, you feel secure in your relationships. You will have at least one or two close, reliable sources of support, and regularly engage in social activities. You are able to love those closest to you without needing to control them. You are also in touch with the capacity to self-love and practice self-care. You will have good boundaries with others, demonstrated by the ability to give without giving yourself away.

When the CARE system is overactive, it becomes difficult to seek enjoyment, fun, and sex. You can get overly concerned with others to your own detriment.

When your CARE system is underactive, you lack the ability to nurture or form lasting social bonds. You are withdrawn from loved ones and may stay removed from any intimate or deep connections. An underactive CARE system will also undermine LUST.

....

#6 PLAY

PLAY is the joyful occupation of all young mammals (and some other lucky critters, too). PLAY is how we learn to explore and experiment with ourselves, each other, and the world, and how we learn to socialize. PLAY is how we rehearse the skills needed to survive and thrive. Mammals learn the skills necessary for everything from hunting to foraging for food to courtship and mating though PLAY. PLAY is how we learn to get along with others, whether we are competing, cooperating, engaging, wooing, or mating — and how we learn who is safe and who should be avoided in such pursuits.

I think of my own two-year-old grandson, who's having a passionate love affair with the world; everything fascinates, everything beckons, everything holds potential for the invention of a new game. For him, eating is play. How many pieces of food can be manipulated and mashed before eaten? How hilarious is it to surreptitiously drop a few carrots onto the floor in anticipation of the dog scampering to steal the treats? The soundtrack to PLAY — joyful laughter, giggles of amusement — in human babies is music to the ears of us caregivers.

Humans are wired by nature to be neotenous, which means we retain certain childlike features and qualities much longer than other animals, with the exception of the other great apes. On average, childhood plus adolescence takes up about 20 percent of our lifespan, although some parents with "grown" kids who fail to launch might argue it takes considerably longer. We have even added a new stage to the human life cycle, the odyssey years, between adolescence and adulthood, encompassing an additional decade of exploration. Becoming a fully developed Homo sapien is a complicated, labor-intensive process. Studies have shown that our frontal lobes — home of the "executive" circuitry underlying our ability to plan, execute complex tasks, and modify our impulsivity — aren't fully functional until we reach our midtwenties. Explains a lot!

While there are several kinds of PLAY, the primordial, wired-in type onto which the others are layered is called rough-and-tumble (RAT — not rat!) play. RAT play is the good old-fashioned roughhousing that for many reasons seems to be going out of style. Part of this reduction in RAT play has to do with parents and schools viewing this kind of behavior as potentially dangerous as well as politically incorrect. We are concerned about bullying or physical injury happening on the playgrounds, thus less time than ever is made available for kids to indulge in this necessary behavior. Indeed, the deficit of RAT play in today's culture seems to be having serious and unintended consequences on the development of our kids. Lacking much needed core RAT playtime, kids' nervous systems are deprived of the activities that will shape and develop the "finely tuned social brain" so necessary for a balanced CARE-PANIC continuum. They don't get feedback on their behaviors as to what people find enjoyable about them or learn the fine art of socializing freestyle. So when they go out into social situations, they freeze. They don't know how to engage, how to be playful interpersonally, or how to burn off energy with and through physical play with others. Panksepp and others believe that children deprived of sufficient opportunities for physical play are at risk for the development of hyperactive urges, distractibility, and restlessness that can easily be construed as symptoms of attention deficit hyperactivity disorders (ADHD). Once diagnosed with ADHD, kids are often prescribed amphetamines, which in turn seem to diminish the urge to play. At the same time, when ADHD has been studied, abundant rough-and-tumble play seems to reduce the severity of the hyperactive symptoms. This is yet another example that, as a culture, we tend to endorse the pharmaceutical solutions that can actually end up discouraging the necessary behavior.

The kinds of play that are more commonly accepted these days involves kids in their rooms hunched over computer screens or devices, in a fantasy world, or involved in one-on-one with an object like a toy or doll. Such play is essentially a solo activity despite other "players" in the room or online. In these types of solo play, from computer games to dolls, the game is played in a world more fantasy than flesh. Our youth are spending way more time in solo and side-by-side parallel play, well beyond the number of years that would otherwise be devoted to face-to-face, interactive, social play. By not engaging in RAT PLAY, kids miss out on the opportunity to learn to coexist with others by creating safe spaces in which to enjoy interaction, and ultimately how to relax our flight and fight stress responses. In this way, PLAY is an important form of learning — both physical and social — that teaches us how to communicate and get along with others; how to enjoy ourselves spontaneously; and how to relax and let go. A healthy working PLAY system is integral to a healthy and robust pleasure system. The PLAY system is literally the source of our social joy chemicals. Our ability to experience pleasure and counter the reverse state of anhedonia is closely tied to rebooting our body-brain connection so that we let ourselves PLAY. It sounds simple, and it is, but it's also a profound human experience and emotion that is necessary for our health and survival.

#6 PLAY

When your PLAY system is in balance, you have a good sense of humor, know how to relax and have fun, and know how to amuse yourself. You have hobbies or interests and otherwise enjoy the zany aspects of life.

When your PLAY system is overactive, you may refuse to engage in mature adult behaviors—think of the perpetual Peter Pans. You may avoid settling down to the business of adulthood and avoid committing to work and partners as you keep searching for more playful pursuits.

When your PLAY system is underactive, you may not be able to relax enough to have fun. If you were unable to play as a child, you may have awkward social skills and have difficulty managing everyday stress. An underactive PLAY system may make you overly self-conscious and controlling.

#7 LUST

Mother Nature has enduringly wired all animals with a primary urge to merge. On one level it appears to be about the survival of the species, but it goes way, way deeper. Putting your genes into the gene pool doesn't directly benefit the individual; it only contributes to the perpetuation of your species, which is why human sexuality is complex — it's not just about reproduction. Sexual behaviors are, at their root, a kind of social glue. The bonds that we make with and through sexual connections forge important affiliations that benefit us. Sexual connections can provide us people and places for safety, people to feed and protect us. It is a way of cementing our bonds and provides transcendent experiences of connection to the self and other. Even looking at the research on animal sexuality, it is clear that social emotions are indeed a key component to LUST. In order to get laid, even animals need some rudimentary social skills. This strong motivation noticeably contributes to the development of social skills across species, in addition to considerable other benefits.

We have tons of data on this that my colleague, mentor, and dear friend, Dr. Beverly Whipple, named one of the fifty most influential scientists in the world by *New Scientist* magazine (2006), compiled in a publication for Planned Parenthood, "The Health Benefits of Sexual Expression." They include physical benefits of sexual activity, such as enhanced overall longevity, reduced risk of coronary heart disease, and decreased risk of type-2 diabetes. Studies also have indicated lower rates of prostate cancer in men tied to more frequent ejaculations, and lowered rates of breast cancers in women who are sexually active. Being sexually active tends to enhance immunity, improve sleep, improve fertility, improve mood, reduce symptoms of anxiety and depression, and help people manage chronic pain. And let's not forget that sexual behavior can enhance feelings of well-being and self-esteem and smooth over rough points in a relationship by facilitating bonding.

And obviously, all the other systems — SEEKING, RAGE, FEAR, PANIC/GRIEF, CARE, and PLAY — all impact LUST. When any of the other emotional systems are out of balance, your LUST will be affected.

....

#7 LUST

When your LUST system is in balance, you experience desire for sex and satisfaction when you have it. You feel comfortable with your desire level and open to exploring ways to experience your pleasure.

When you LUST system is overactive, you may show some form of out-of-control, inappropriate, or harmful sexual behavior. For instance, you might get overinvolved with pornography or masturbate excessively.

When your LUST system is underactive, you have little interest in sex and cannot feel sexual desire.

....

When any one of our core emotional systems becomes imbalanced — as is the case when we are anxious or anhedonic or feel sexually frustrated — our top brain cannot function to its capacity; the primary emotional system of the bottom of the brain and secondary level of the mind/brain are in charge, driving you. That's why no amount of wishful thinking can move you out of an anxious state, or help you feel the thrill of sexual excitement, or move you to tears of joy, unless you become aware of what's up in the basement of your brain. Our higher-level minds just aren't up to the task of turning around the battleship of raw affects sensitized by old experiences and emotional habits. No matter how hard we work our PFC, we simply can't seem able to restore ourselves back to the pleasures nature intended.

Our core emotional lives affect us more than we have acknowledged in current psychology. Although we pay so much attention now to "top-down" processes and higher-level learning, we absolutely need to cue into the bottom-up processing that lies beneath and fuses our experience of living and loving. What's fascinating, to my mind, is that this level of emotional experience is still by and large often nonconscious. What we mean by conscious is really a small window of approximately twenty to thirty seconds. Ultimately, we live in that small window of what is "working memory," yet so much more is happening "under the hood."

One of Panksepp's most important contributions is his suggestion that it's only in seeing how our basic, more primal emotions function that we can then appreciate and in turn control (manipulate) our own experience. In other words, at our most basic level, unless these core levels of emotion are working well for us, our PFC won't really have any leverage. Further, without adequately addressing the core levels of "raw" emotion, our attempts to regulate them through treatments that focus on cognitions (thoughts, insights, or beliefs) — even in conjunction with behavioral therapies — simply may not be sufficient to produce sustainable benefits. We know that despite our best intentions, our keenest insights, and our most determined efforts to modify problematic ways of thinking and behaving, we all too often drift back to the very states of distress we seek to change.

Despite the evidence that Panksepp, Darwin, and others have provided about these innate emotional capacities, we are only now becoming focused on extending our clinical knowledge of how to positively impact them.

As you will see in part 2, when I introduce people from my practice, imbalances in any of the seven core emotions can have a huge impact on our overall well-being. When any of these is disrupted or undermined, people not only experience difficulty experiencing pleasure — sexual or otherwise — but they suffer from an unshakable unease or unhappiness.

For these reasons and more, our "animal instincts" are not to be ignored, but rather used as intelligent information to address anhedonia and make true change. There is a huge difference between being informed by these feelings and being hijacked by them. The ability to avoid this emotional hijacking is key to regaining happier, healthier lives.

Part Two

......

Restoring the Emotional Brain

4

Rebalancing Your SEEKING System: Liking What You Need

At nineteen years old, Tim is one of my youngest clients. He lives at home with his parents, does not work, and is too afraid to venture out in the world. His parents are worried that after graduating from high school two years ago, where he did so well, Tim can't seem to do anything. "He just sits on the couch in the den watching TV, playing video games, and reading." The good news is that after two weeks of hounding from his parents, Tim came to my office, and he's been coming for the past few weeks, gradually warming up to me and becoming more engaged.

Tim is a slim, tall, pleasant-looking kid, the kind that wouldn't stick out in a crowd. He spends most of each session looking at his sneakers. When he periodically looks up long enough to meet my gaze, I am wowed by the color of his eyes. Sky blue. Baby blue. Paul Newman blue. But what truly blows my mind is the sadness in them. Even though he generally looks younger than his age, the eyes that gaze back are those of an old and very melancholic soul.

He says that he feels okay, but that his parents want him in therapy because they think he is wasting his life. Tim appears to be stuck in a failure-to-launch loop that has tied him up since he graduated high school. He begins to fill me in. Right after graduation, he tried a brief stint at the local community college but stopped going to classes because he didn't see the point. His parents, both successful midlevel managers, keep encouraging him to try a different school. Although he tells them he will apply elsewhere, he doesn't. He has a part-time job at a pizza parlor, and he likes to draw, specifically cartooning. He spends tons of time gaming, watching sports, drawing in his room, and occasionally hanging out with his younger brother, age seventeen. But even still, Tim spends most of his time alone.

I ask Tim whether he's lonely and if he wants to date. He shrugs and tells me he doesn't know if he's lonely. About the dating, he says he feels too awkward. As we develop more of a rapport, he fesses up. "I just feel too self-conscious when I am around girls," he reflects. Digging deeper, Tim reveals that he has a tendency to "feel panicky" when he is in crowds, in classes, at restaurants, eating in front of people, and sometimes even for "no reason at all."

No one really knows this fact about Tim. It isn't exactly cool for a young man to expose a panicky nature to peers or family. Sure, his parents know something isn't quite right — that he is a bit avoidant. His teachers saw him as a quiet, shy kid. His brother and the neighborhood kids think he is quirky. And since he hasn't had a full-blown panic attack that would call attention to his problem, he has managed his symptoms so far by laying low and avoiding people, places, and situations that would trigger it. Sticking close to home where he feels safely attached to the family is both an attempt at a solution and, unbeknownst to Tim, the perpetuation of the problem as it prevents him from developing more confidence through experience.

And although he is not depressed (yet), it's clear that his PANIC/ GRIEF system is interfering with — if not suppressing — his SEEKING system. Showing up to therapy is the first conscious step he has taken recently to activate this SEEKING system, so that's a good sign. He absolutely needs this motivation to come online, so to speak, so that his appetite and curiosity will return and serve as an antidote to his genetic propensity for PANIC/GRIEF. If he doesn't learn how to fire up his SEEKING system, he runs the risk of becoming increasingly panicked as he isolates and avoids social contacts — the real face-to-face and one-to-one social and sexual enjoyment a young person needs for growth and joy.

Bringing Tim's SEEKING System into Balance

At first, Tim's therapy focuses on me asking him questions — for instance, "Are you completely satisfied with life in the den?" I am trying to whet his appetite for a girlfriend, companionship, a career, a curiosity in what interests him. And as I always do with clients, I ask him about his sexuality, just like everything else. Have you explored yourself sexually? With clients my rule of thumb is that if you can talk about sex, you can talk about everything! As a therapist and neuroscientist, I know that real change can only occur if I understand a person in their totality, and that includes how sex figures in their life. It's equally important for Tim to understand himself from a sexual point of view — it's an unfettered view right into the center of his core emotional self that will help later on when we do more top-down work. Right now, though, I know that Tim needs to start by receiving permission to tap into all that he wants, sex included.

Tim's responses to my questions are illuminating: he admits that underneath his nervousness, which he tries to control by staying inside and close to his family, he harbors a concrete fear of his sexual desires. For no apparent reason, Tim has come to fear that his desire to kiss, touch, and be with a girl will end in catastrophe — either with a girl rejecting him or showing outright disgust. He keeps playing scenarios in his head that have come to be like a live-action loop when he goes to bed each night. The intensity of this fantasy has made him so fearful that, in defense mode, he has shut down all other feelings, flattening him out.

The first level of helping Tim begins by acknowledging how his SEEKING system has flattened and then helping him become aware of what he wants — a girlfriend, a job, a social life, for example. Of course, I am wondering what's underneath. Why does he seem like he has given up wanting anything for himself? What has happened to his curiosity? His enthusiasm for things that bring him pleasure? Why has he stopped SEEKING?

For Tim, he consciously and unconsciously shut down his SEEKING system as a defensive measure to contain his PANIC/GRIEF; indeed, if he were not already wired this way, his SEEKING system might have been sufficient to overcome his fears of being sexual. As it was, however, he couldn't get out of the FEAR loop he was feeling. And, though we can't rewire him, the best way to get him out of defense mode (triggered by his fear) is by stoking his SEEKING system.

How the Brain Learns: SEEKING Pleasure

If sex is essentially rewarding because of the pleasure it brings, then why do we avoid having sex? Why does sex become painful? A cause of anxiety and trepidation?

Historically, neuroscientists, cognitive psychologists, and other researchers who have studied the brain and human behavior described the SEEKING system as the "reward" system or pathway. Although the SEEKING system is very much related to reward, or more accurately reinforcement, our current understanding of how it works is much more nuanced. The way our brain is designed, we are hardwired to *want* all sorts of rewards (from food, to physical stimuli, to gratification from a job well done) — and this wanting (one dimension of the reward system) acts more or less automatically and relies on the lower brain. As our desire for more complex rewards develops, we recruit more of our cognitive capacities that operate from the "high" brain. Indeed, our capacity to experience pleasure starts with SEEKING and ends with learning. These distinctions are echoed by the history of experimentation surrounding the reward processes.

Beginning with the early behaviorists, scientists thought that reward processing was simply an expression of how our brain learns (i.e., the outcome of a built-in mechanism to go after rewards, and once procured, the reward reinforces the behavior). Edward Thorndike, who identified a more complex form of learning that he called operant conditioning, conducted experiments in which he observed a cat in a cage. When the cat made attempts through trial and error that allowed it to get out of the cage and eat, the cat then repeated this action each time it was put in the cage. The cat's behaviors "operated" on the environment, creating a desired consequence — his escaping the cage in order to find a treat.

What emerged from this line of early experiments was how rewards figure into the way we learn. This evolution in our understanding began in large part with the work of James Olds and Peter Milner, who serendipitously discovered the "reward circuits" while studying other brain regions. They went on to do a series of experiments in which they attached electrodes to various regions of the brains of rats to see how they would respond to pleasurable electrical stimulation. The animals pressed levers to obtain the stimulation. What surprised Olds and Milner was their observation that animals got so caught up in pressing the levers to obtain the stimulation, they forgot to eat and drink. Olds and Milner had stumbled upon two important discoveries: 1) the "hot spots" for pleasure were located in numerous locations, not just one as previously thought; 2) that dopamine neurons located in the midbrain played an active role in whatever was going on to motivate the animals to press the lever — a response so strong they stopped eating and drinking for a while. Later, scientists observed that these spikes in dopamine occurred not only when the animal obtained the electrical stimulation (the reward) but also when they *predicted* they were going to get the reward of either electric stimulation or, alternatively, a delicious juice treat.

Underlying the motivation to obtain pleasure is our brain's prediction or expectation of a pleasurable reward. In fact, the pathway to pleasure has been defined as having three distinct components, each with its own neurobiological mechanism and each representing a kind of phase in a sequence. First, the initiation is marked by a *wanting* of pleasure; followed by a *liking* of what was sought after (a kind of consummation); followed then by a *learning*. This last piece of the sequence ensures that the brain-body remembers the connection between the wanting and the liking and encodes this connection in the midlevel of the brain, enabling the prediction of reward in the future.

Most of this process is enabled by mesolimbic dopamine that operates from the midbrain. Mesolimbic dopamine primes motivation, attention, and expectation — all features of the SEEKING system. This dopaminergic system is essentially a "reinforcement pathway" that stems from localized subcortical regions of the brain that form "hedonic hot spots" that reinforce positive experiences so that we remember them. This type of memory can bypass higher-order brain areas, including the PFC; it stays subconscious (i.e., in the limbic system).

When in good working order, the SEEKING system is supposed to function like this: i) our brain seeks a pleasant stimulus; ii) it then computes the reward value and associated costs; iii) it determines effort requirements to obtain that stimulus; iv) it decides to obtain that stim-

ulus; and v) it anticipates and increases motivation to obtain that stimulus. Dopamine is the primary neurochemical that "pushes" this chain
reaction.

For years, up through much of the 1980s, scientists thought that
the dopamine spikes actually generated or enabled the pleasure from
the stimuli — this is why people often call dopamine the pleasure neurotransmitter. But more recently, neuroscientists have teased apart all of
what's going on with this process of reward learning. Though dopamine
levels have also been shown to correlate with the transition from wanting
(the desire for pleasure) to liking (i.e., the experience of pleasure), it is
not what enables people to experience the sensation of liking.

At first, when we go from wanting a reward (incentive salience) and
then obtain the reward, experiencing pleasurable stimuli, phasic dopamine spikes. Right after, the dopamine transfers back a signal to the midlevel (learning/memory) brain, thereby creating an association with the
reward, enabling the prediction of the reward in the future. However, if
we continue to get the same reward, the dopamine spike lessens and the
learning ceases.

Think about Tim for a moment: if he wasn't wired to be nervous, he
would have more than likely acted on his interest in girls and desire to
be sexual by being more actively social. This SEEKING behavior would
have calmed down his PANIC (had it not been so strongly wired in) and
prevented him from going into total defense mode (shutdown). Even
talking to a girl would have the positive potential to spike his dopamine
and reinforce the pleasure pathway enough to motivate him to repeat the
behavior if his PANIC/GRIEF system weren't so hair triggered). When
the wanting and the reward are encoded, then each time Tim talked with
a girl, he could experience a reinforcing spike of dopamine. This could
even happen when he simply recalled talking to a girl. But alas, Tim's
PANIC/GRIEF system, as is, gets in his way.

This relationship between wanting and SEEKING, the hallmark of the dopaminergic system, is more complicated yet — and has most recently been described more like an instance of learning than really one of reward. As Wolfram Schultz, one of the pre-eminent scientists studying reward says, "rewards produce learning."

However, he and others have pointed out that this kind of reward learning only continues if there's a *difference* between expectation of reward and the actual reward. Our brains need some kind of difference between the actual reward procured (positive or negative) and the expectation in order to record the learning. This kind of learning is also referred to as temporal difference. As Schultz puts it: "if the reward is exactly as predicted . . . there is no prediction error, and we keep our prediction and behavior unchanged; we learn nothing . . . The whole learning mechanism works because we want positive prediction errors and hate negative prediction errors . . . This is what drives life and evolution." Expectations also play a huge role in our emotions. When we get what we want — and what we expect — we are pretty happy — at least for a while. However, we can quickly habituate to getting the same reward over and over. We end up wanting something new or something more. If we get more than we expect, we are happy again (for a while). On the other hand, when our expectations for what we want are violated negatively (we don't get what we expect), we can get pretty pissed off. To put it simply: the violation of our expectations, for better or worse, are often the source of our emotional reactions.

There are two types of dopamine at play in learning that comes from prediction error — phasic and tonic dopamine — and the interplay of the two sheds further light on the complexity of the SEEKING system and how it's supposed to work. When a pleasurable reward is predicted, phasic dopamine is released by an automatic process in the lower brain. Tonic dopamine (released and regulated by the PFC) refers to that "background" dopamine that "floats" around, trying to help regulate the firing of the phasic dopamine. The brain-body is in a near-constant enterprise of maintaining a balance between these seemingly opposite dopamine actions. When our SEEKING system is functioning normally, phasic dopamine regulates our motivation to go after pleasant sensations and stay away from unpleasant sensations or stimuli. If phasic dopamine is underactive, we have a low response to stimulation; if it's overactive, it can cause impulsive or out-of-control SEEKING. In both cases, it's tonic dopamine's job to keep phasic dopamine in working order.

However, some people are genetically predisposed to have low levels of tonic dopamine, like Tim, or may have fewer dopamine receptors where the neurotransmitter can do its job, making them more susceptible to both depression or the flatlining of anhedonia and/or not being able to regulate the firing response of phasic dopamine. Indeed, Tim is working at a deficit of dopamine; biochemically, it is probably that he either is missing some dopamine receptors or doesn't produce enough; as a result, his brain-body is flooded with stress hormones that make him avoid social situations. Anyone who has gone through a prolonged period of stress will ramp up his/her tonic dopamine levels, which ultimately obscure the effects of phasic dopamine, altering the person's SEEKING system. And what this can ultimately do is create a state of depletion such that anhedonia becomes the emotional wallpaper that we are so habituated to that we don't even notice that what is lacking is our ability to experience fulfilling, satisfying pleasures.

And in the case of Tim, who hasn't been experiencing the spike from SEEKING (phasic), but rather an absence of wanting altogether, his baseline tonic further inhibits his brain-body system, hence his sticking to the couch in the den. In his case, we need to help him stir the initial desire, the wanting for more sensation at its most basic level to help rebalance his dopamine levels. The fact that dopamine itself is more complicated than once thought reinforces the idea that we can experience disruptions in the SEEKING system in more than one way—not enough tonic dopamine floating in the "background"; not enough receptors to warrant strong "bursts" of phasic dopamine with a predicted reward; or too much tonic dopamine, undermining the intensity of the phasic spikes.

Some aspects of this pleasure cycle are conscious, but most are nonconscious and happen below the level of our awareness. What's significant is that this cycle occurs similarly in all mammals—humans and nonhumans alike—suggesting/indicating that this evolutionarily old path or cycle of pleasure evolved because it has a clear survival function.

The fact that pleasure is not simply a desire for a pleasing reward but also has important biologic functions is fascinating—indeed, I think it points both to how we might get unstuck from anhedonia but also why sex, in particular, is so important in all of this. In other words, as a mindful yet somatic experience, sex has the capacity to elicit the pleasure pathway and reboot the SEEKING system, jolting us out of anhedonia. I feel certain that if Tim comes to see himself as a finely tuned Maserati that needs more maintenance than the average pickup truck and gains control of gradually opening up the SEEKING system step by step—inch by inch—he will learn how to harness his nervous system and emerge from the den. So Tim's problem is not sexual in nature—but arose from his dysregulated SEEKING system.

....

The underlying neurobiology reveals that people with a disrupted SEEKING system are unable to:

- Anticipate or predict reward

- Associate value or cost of reward

- Determine effort required for reward

- Integrate information to make a decision

- Become motivated to perform or act

···

Stoking the SEEKING System and Discovering Your Desire Curve

Regardless of the causes of anhedonia, when the SEEKING system is out of balance, it's usually disrupted in two typical ways: it's either in overdrive like we saw with Matt, discussed in chapter one, or is underactive, as in the case of Tim. Matt's SEEKING system is clearly in overdrive: stuck in a cycle of wanting with no liking. Acting as if out of control, Matt continually sought sexual encounters and stimulation but without ever having the satisfaction that comes with liking what he was after. His dopaminergic pathway (his reinforcement pathway) did not offer him enough satisfying dopamine to sustain a pleasurable response and didn't hang around long enough to develop sustainable feelings of CARE and bonding, which would have offered him deeper satisfaction from the opioids. The stress of his lifestyle further disrupted his dopamine functioning, keeping him stuck in SEEKING. When the lower brain is thus affected, it can't experience the satisfying bump up of functioning phasic dopamine on its own to stay in balance; the midbrain's patterns of behavior then take over and reinforce behaviors that continue to undermine the dysregulation.

With addiction, an individual has to consciously (very high awareness) address the exponential seeking and striving in order to override the tendency that has now become automatic. The strength of the dopamine cry for the opiate receptors keeps a person who is addicted hyperfocused on one thing: that fix. And no fix is big enough. People who are addicted to gambling, food, sex, alcohol, or drugs share this same dysregulation — their neuromodulators are out of whack, which further reinforces neural patterns of behavior and emotion that are exceptionally difficult to interrupt. Think of the actor Robert Downey Jr., who was once asked during his bad boy druggie days what his favorite drug was. His answer was simply "more." For people struggling with addiction, the spikes of dopamine continue to go up and up without learning because their reward system is no longer working the way it's supposed to.

But is Matt suffering from sex addiction? No. Matt is not an addict. Matt is responding to the current cultural zeitgeist of dating apps — the ease of access to sex has exacerbated his drive to seek. And because his other affiliative emotions are not online, they cannot balance the out-of-whack SEEKING system. If, however, Matt does begin to tap into these affiliative emotions — CARE and PLAY in particular — his SEEKING system will naturally come into balance. He will become present enough to seek partners with whom he can connect and begin to slow down the constant SEEKING behavior and learn to stop and experience the plea-sure, the satisfaction.

The other recognizable and common way that a dysregulated SEEK-ING system shows up is when SEEKING is underactive, and people emotionally flatline, like Tim. They experience no exuberance, no en-ergy, no curiosity, no willingness to explore. This kind of flat affect is associated with a tendency toward depression, though it surely does not completely explain a very complex disease. A flatlining level of energy is an indicator that your SEEKING system needs a boost — it's depleted, or otherwise something in the dopaminergic pathway is being disrupted.

A downregulated SEEKING system can squash LUST for other rea-sons as well. One of my clients, Yvonne, is worried at thirty-six that she has fallen out of love with her husband, Paul. "I used to love having sex with him; now I have zero motivation." Paul is becoming frustrated and resentful. She "goes through the motions" but her "heart isn't in it." When I ask her if it's just sex that's being affected, she tells me, "Pretty much."

After a few sessions of getting to know her and some of her history, I learn that this flatlining of hers began about three years into their marriage. At first, she was able to "get in the mood" by running (activating endorphins and endocannabinoids) and working hard in her studio (she's an artist and feels pleasure when she paints). "Sex was still something I wanted, looked forward to. But now," she tells me, she's "avoiding these activities" and doesn't "even have desire to find pleasures outside of the bedroom — not even giving them a chance."

I then explain to Yvonne that she's being a bit hard on herself. It's absolutely normal to lose some of your spontaneous desire after a romance begins to become more familiar. And as the novelty of any relationship will inevitably wear off, both the SEEKING system and the LUST system begin to reset to more of a baseline state.

This loss of spontaneous desire is incredibly common for women and also for some men. But what Yvonne was also not aware of are the very real gender differences between men and women: the makeup of female sex hormones and male sex hormones are different and act in different ways in the brain. In a nutshell, males have more sex on the brain than females, and this shows up as "wanting" more sex. Though both partners may have been experiencing a loss of spontaneous desire, Yvonne was feeling it more acutely, likely because she is a woman. Women often have to "work" harder to light up their LUST — that's why PLAY and connection are so important to have in the mix to offset the inevitable ebbing of spontaneous desire that accompanies what I call new relationship energy (NRE).

Regardless of who is experiencing the LUST fallout, the ebbing of desire is often exacerbated because women and men misunderstand what's going on in the relationship. Instead of seeing the fall off of LUST as a natural downregulation of both SEEKING and LUST systems, people will assume that "they're out of love" or "no longer attracted" to their partner. They can also, like Yvonne, blame themselves.

But the lust isn't gone; it's just returned to its preromance baseline, its set point.

All of us have a baseline of desire and experience what I call a "desire curve" that fluctuates throughout our lives. (In chapter 8, you will delve more into both your desire curve, which will help you understand your set point, and your NRE, which signifies the high of spontaneous desire that accompanies new romances; for now, check out the exercise below to understand, for instance, how sex positive you are, how past experiences may be affecting your LUST system, or how your other core systems might be suppressing your lust. Chronic stress, trauma, and other biopsychosocial factors can inhibit SEEKING and LUST.)

For Yvonne, she first needs to understand what that baseline is so that she can stop blaming herself. And then, she needs to figure out ways to jump-start her LUST and SEEKING systems through physical arousal. In recounting her sex history, she is able to get a sense of her preromance sexual baseline and how she typically experiences sexual desire outside of or before a new romantic relationship. Again, a waning of desire after the first several months to a year of a new relationship is common — but in this case, the drop-off was more severe — probably because her other go-to pleasurable activities like running, painting, and yoga were not sustaining a pumped-up SEEKING system. She had become too depleted of PLAY and joy.

With this new awareness, Yvonne begins to relax and stops judging herself so harshly. She also begins to play with a few of the Good Sex Tools to help her harness and mobilize her SEEKING system and lead to real, pleasurable solutions. From my perspective, Yvonne's situation is actually quite simple: when she recognizes that backing away from what she loves to do — what arouses and feeds her curiosity and enthusiasm — is hindering her, she is able to rechannel that energy back into her relationship. And she stops feeling guilty.

....

Good Sex Tool: Your Desire Curve

In order to accurately assess the intensity of your own sexual desire, as well as the sexual vibe of your relationship (if you're in one), it's crucial that you understand your own sexual temperament, which is the basis of your desire curve, that arc of sexual desire that includes both your highs and lows of desire, as well as the plateaus. In order to cue into your sexual temperament, take these steps:

1. Think back to the level of sexual desire you had before your current relationship on a scale of 1 to 10 (10 being the highest/most often):

    a. How often did you think about sex at all?
    b. How often did you masturbate?
    c. How often did you fantasize about sex?
    d. How often did you actually have sex (if you did at all)?

This number is an estimate of your baseline of Sexual Desire.

2. Next, repeat the above steps related to when you were first in your current relationship. This is the time when you and your partner were just getting to know each other, when sex was at the forefront of your minds . . . and bodies. On a scale of 1 to 10 (10 being the highest/ most often):

   a. How often did you think about sex at all?

   b. How often did you masturbate?

   c. How often did you fantasize about sex?

   d. How often did you actually have sex (if you did at all)?

This number is your new relationship energy (NRE) score.

3. Now, compare your current level of sexual interest and desire to the baseline prior to your current relationship — not to the NRE levels. On a scale of 1 to 10 (10 being the highest/most often):

   a. How often do you think about sex at all?

   b. How often do you masturbate?

   c. How often do you fantasize about sex?

   d. How often do you actually have sex (if you do at all)?

Some people actually sink lower than their baseline, post-NRE. This drop-off may be due to environmental or situational factors, including health, hormones, exercise (a lack thereof), stress, anxiety, boredom, changes in life circumstances, or financial changes.

··

··

Good Sex Tool: Check Your SEEKING System

- How curious are you to learn new things?

- Are you open to trying new positions?

- When you have sex with yourself or your partner, do you tend to do the same thing?

- If you've lost interest in sex, can you pinpoint when this occurred? Was it a gradual process or did it happen suddenly?

- How would you describe your sexual set point (i.e., your baseline interest in sex)?

....

The SEEKING system has a powerful impact on our entire network of core emotional systems. It's always a good place to start when you notice that you are not feeling as motivated as usual or you are racing around, unable to stop moving, chasing, or SEEKING. As we will explore in the next chapter, when the SEEKING system is out of balance, the defensive emotional systems are usually out of balance—heightened FEAR, reactivity, difficulty containing RAGE, and/or easily triggered PANIC/GRIEF mode. An out-of-whack SEEKING system has an analogous impact on our affiliative systems: LUST, CARE, and PLAY are dampened, further keeping us in an anhedonic rut.

Sometimes it's the other way around: if you've experienced a traumatic event that has overactivated your FEAR response, for example, your SEEKING system will get suppressed. Who can feel curious about novelty when they are petrified for their safety?

The good news is that in all of these cases, you can reverse anhedonia and restoke the SEEKING system. When your SEEKING system is revving again—neither over- or underactive—you will feel energetic, curious, motivated, and excited about life. And as the stories of Tim and Yvonne suggest, sex can get you there.

5

Hot-Tempered and Afraid: Taming Our Defenses

K atie is a thirty-seven-year-old mother of three who has never, ever had an orgasm. A slim, statuesque Irish American with huge brown eyes and a cascade of wavy auburn hair, she is a human re sources executive at a large company and sought my help for her inability to orgasm, what sex therapists diagnose as primary anorgasmia. From a biological perspective, Katie is an extremely fit, healthy woman in the prime of her life. There is no indication of any medical issues or hormonal imbalances. And since she says she doesn't experience any significant depression or anxiety and has never been in therapy before, it's clear there's another reason behind her inability to orgasm. Curiously, Katie says that other than being frustrated about not being able to orgasm, she very much enjoys sex. She has lots of spontaneous sexual desire, lubricates easily, and experiences sexual activity as a positive bonding experience with her new husband. So, if all of this is working, why can't she orgasm?

When FEAR Hijacks LUST

Katie is not only frustrated with herself, she also feels deep shame about not being able to orgasm. And like many women in her position, she believes that there is something wrong with her and that this so-called disorder says something about her as a woman and a wife.

"I feel inferior to other women — like I am less than they are and am lacking something important. And this issue undermines my general sense of self-confidence. In fact, I think I am a bit of a perfectionist as a result of this one thing I can't do. I have to try harder and accomplish more to make up for my inadequacy. My mind is busy nearly all of the time."

When I ask Katie to explain how sex feels with her husband, she says, "When we start making love, I immediately become self-conscious and start obsessing. Instead of relaxing, instead of being there, having the experience, I go into my head. As soon as the sensations start building up, I get excited and start thinking about whether this might just be the one time I actually am able to orgasm, and then — kaput — it's over before it started. And there were a bunch of times when I felt like the sensations were getting really intense, and I think I shut them down. It's like when I tried skiing a couple of times and couldn't learn how because as soon as I start moving a bit fast downhill, I would throw myself down. It feels like fear to me. I think I am afraid of losing control."

Katie's anorgasmia was a significant factor in the breakup of her first marriage. Her husband was her high school sweetheart and the father of her three children. "We didn't really discuss this issue. We both went to Catholic school and were pretty traditional about sex. He tried. We tried. I know it frustrated my ex-husband that he couldn't make me have an orgasm. He was my first lover, of course. We thought it would just take time. He felt inadequate, like it was his fault. Then he seemed to give up and just go for his own pleasure. Like he had lost hope. I do think he ended up thinking there was something wrong with me. Once I asked him whether he thought I should try to masturbate, since I had read somewhere that it might help, and he looked at me like I was nuts. That probably reinforced my feelings that masturbation was creepy and dirty for women. And over the eight years we were married, sex became more infrequent and we grew apart. We didn't really fight. We just stopped talking and became more like roommates. He traveled for work and I was busy with the kids. When we had the twins, we pretty much stopped having sex altogether."

Katie's second husband, on the other hand, is more open minded — he is actually the one who encouraged Katie to find a sex therapist. "You deserve to have orgasms, too," he observed. Katie reports that unlike her first husband, who took this all very personally, her new partner "doesn't make this about him." It's clearly his support that has given her the courage to find some answers.

On the surface, Katie is open to sex, enjoys it, and seems to be generally sex positive. She is sophisticated and nonjudgmental of others — but does seem to be putting a lot of pressure on herself. She believes that she might have inherited a "gene" or some other predisposing factor that makes her incapable of having an orgasm. Why does she think this? Her fifty-eight-year-old mother confided her own anorgasmia to her during an uncharacteristically candid talk they had when Katie's first marriage was in the process of crashing and burning. When asked about her sexual history, Katie reports that she has had a total of two lovers, both of whom became husbands. When I ask about how she learned about sex, Katie winces.

"No one really discussed this with me. All health class in school taught us was about abstinence and things like menstruation. Later on, I read a book my cousin gave me. She was a bit older, and her parents were hippies. They talked about sex. I thought it was strange since in my house that topic was totally off limits. We weren't even allowed to watch PG-13 movies. It just wasn't done."

The absence of discussion in her own home signaled to Katie that sex was not okay and that it carried with it shame and judgment. As she and I begin to talk through her early associations with sex, she begins to remember what she had learned not only from her mother but also from the girls and teachers (some of whom were nuns) at Catholic school. The explicit information about sex was scant, but the implicit messages were clear and deeply felt: Sex is scary. Sex is dirty. Good girls just don't do it. The sex and fear connection became well established.

Remember how the midlevel mind holds on to learning that comes along with strong core emotional states? And how these early "learnings" stay with us but are often not accurate? What I infer from all of what Katie is describing is this: Katie had tons of conditioning at Catholic school that good girls simply didn't have sex — either with other people, or themselves.

During one of our first conversations, Katie recalls an incident. "Geez, I haven't thought about this in years. When I was seven or eight years old, I was taking a bath and the soap slipped between my legs. And when I reached down to find it, I touched myself down there and it felt good. While I was touching myself, my mom happened to walk in. She started yelling at me, 'You must never do that, do you understand?' My mom had really never yelled at me and so I felt awful. Dirty. Ashamed. And we never discussed that afterwards. Never."

What is the core emotion behind the learned feeling of shame? FEAR. Shame is induced in us as a higher-level mechanism to keep us "safe" by steering us clear of being ostracized from our supports — a fate that endangers our survival, be it physical or psychological. As a result, as is the case with Katie, access to the LUST system becomes very conditional. At the top of her brain, she can feel positive toward sex, but underneath, in the basement of her brain, the original FEAR is locking up her body — to such a degree that she cannot orgasm. The FEAR system becomes so overly activated that though she thinks she wants to let go into having orgasmic sex (in her higher-level brain), her midlevel brain has her in its clutches. Indeed, her LUST system has absorbed the old messages about sex and old experiences that were upsetting, infusing her emotional systems and stifling her full release into sexuality.

For Katie, similar to Tim, FEAR is a powerful constraint to LUST.

The FEARful Brain

Approximately forty million Americans, about 18 percent of the population, are diagnosed with an anxiety disorder. This anxiety, other than being a reflection of pervasive anhedonia, is also a reflection of brains that have become overridden by fear — in other words, the FEAR system has become hijacked.

Our fear response, which is located very near the pain pathway, incorporates the periaqueductal gray (PAG), a midbrain structure made up of gray matter. The FEAR system wiring goes directly from the PAG to the amygdala and then back again. As you may remember, the amygdala is very much involved in processing both emotions and memories (via inputs to its neighbor, the hippocampus). It also plays a role in the emotional nuances of decision making. One way I've come to think of the amygdala is like a big biological highlighter calling our attention to very good or very bad events, experiences, or feelings with utmost urgency, influencing what is important to remember. This emotional signaling system tells us that something is very important (based on the valence of the stimuli — good or bad — and its intensity) and flags information that has potential emotional and or physical consequences. But an amygdala that is hot-wired with fear makes someone hypervigilant; at the level of the brain, the attention system is hijacked, and we become unable to turn down or turn off the FEAR system. Damage to our amygdala, for instance, prevents an appropriate experience of FEAR, as well as the inability to learn from negative consequences. Either extreme could potentially sabotage our ability to experience pleasure and contentment.

Think of Katie: her mother's angry and shame-inducing response to Katie's early sexual exploration was so strong that it created a very powerful fear response in Katie. And since the FEAR system has most likely evolved to promote fast and furious learning about the specifics of what we experience as painful (an angry response from our mothers, for instance) and promote the kind of learning that keeps us away from harm, Katie is being held back by a now maladaptive defensive reaction. Her amygdala prompted her memory system to encode this experience, creating an automatic connection between anything sexual and that old learned fear response to her mother's reaction to Katie's touching her own genitals. Because these core emotions live in the bottom brain, they are lodged deeply in our unconscious memory banks and continue to exert influence on us until we become aware of them. For Katie, her fear grew into the hypervigilance that is now preventing her from orgasming. In Tim's case, his fear response was a defensive reaction to help him cope with his tendency toward panic (out of control nervousness). FEAR is stubborn and it can easily block LUST.

Regaining Control over FEAR in Sex

So how does Katie's embedded fear response get untangled from her capacity to orgasm? After our initial discussion, it became clear that Katie needed to learn how to play her own sexual instrument (practice masturbation) in order to "invite her orgasm to find her" before she would be likely to experience orgasm with a partner. This is a common next step for women who have not explored their own sexuality or masturbated successfully. They need to lay down their own orgasm pathways. All kinds of learning, whether it be motor (physical) skills or cognitive abilities, is a form of change or adaptation that depends on strengthening the connections between the cells of the nervous system. Katie literally needs to establish the connections between her genitals and her brain pathways to experience sensation, pleasure, and ultimately learn to have an orgasm. I advise her to seek out information about masturbation from a number of sources and order a Magic Wand vibrator — this will help her get intense results and reinforce her orgasmic pathways. I also explain that it may take some time — for most women, masturbation takes some practice. It is more than likely that her orgasm will unfold over time, as she strengthens the connections within her own sexual pathways. Keep stimulating your genitals and the pathways to your orgasm brain will appear.

When Katie returns a week or so later, she reports that she had indeed gotten the vibrator, but had not done the masturbation exploration. I ask her to be curious (i.e., stimulate her SEEKING system) about what was in the way.

"I just don't feel like being sexual with myself. I need to connect with my husband in order to feel sexy."

Although Katie had complied with getting the vibrator, she only used it once — during sex with her husband. "It felt good, really intense. My husband encouraged me to play with myself during foreplay, but I didn't orgasm and I haven't gotten around to masturbation."

This one step, though in the right direction, reveals that Katie's sex negative conditioning still appears to be blocking her from doing what her top-level mind consciously wants — to learn how to orgasm.

What Katie needs is to create new positive experiences to override the old, negative (midlevel brain) associations, which requires that she feel safe and relaxed so that she can calm down her FEAR system and learn that sex is okay. She also needs to tap into her top-level brain processing and make a conscious change in how she envisions the outcome of this work. I share with her an exercise called "Reframing Your Outcomes" (see below) that many of my clients begin with; it is a powerful tool that enables you to move from a "problem" frame ("I can't orgasm") to an "outcome" frame ("I will learn to orgasm").

What pushes these new learnings and ultimately transforms her relationship with her own sexuality is an experiential activity that will update her associations in an immediate, positive way. Together, we watch a very explicit instructional video about the coital alignment technique, a specialized version of the missionary position developed to help women more easily orgasm from intercourse. The video shows three young, beautiful couples in turn demonstrating variants of the technique — having hot, juicy intercourse along with tons of pleasure. While watching the video, Katie begins to laugh so hard, she cries. She is discharging old distress and shame. She leaves the session glowing. The laughter and the play-filled release has the power to wipe away the residual shame and negative associations — it's orgasmic in and of itself.

Two weeks later, Katie calls to report that during a business trip, she used the vibrator while having phone sex with her husband and had a big fat orgasm — her first orgasm ever! Then she went home and found that she could do it again — and again — through masturbation and also with her husband orally stimulating her. Katie had learned a powerful lesson: that it was up to her to take charge of her own sexuality and accept that most women do not orgasm through intercourse alone. Katie was fortunate. She was able to quickly release old fears and the related shame. Not everyone can move through old defenses so swiftly.

FEAR can be tricky — especially early, powerful associations that get locked into our unconscious (midlevel) memories. They are stubborn defensive mechanisms that are difficult — but not impossible — to root out. Let's take a look at another defensive system and how it can inhibit sexual experience and pleasure in general.

....

Good Sex Tool: Reframing Your Outcomes

Once you bring your body into an open and relaxed place, calming your emotional system, it's time to do some top-down reframing so that you can reignite your pleasure circuit and consciously connect with yourself or your partner. This powerful tool is an adaption of a classic neurolinguistic programming (NLP) exercise that shows you how to switch from a "problem" frame to a more empowering "outcome" approach. Transformation begins with getting clear on what you want to create in the first place.

Here's how it works.

- First, think about something that has been really bugging you, an issue that is problematic, stressful, or otherwise unpleasant.

- Now ask yourself the following questions: Why can't I fix or solve this issue? What's wrong with me, or the other person (if it involves a relationship), or the situation that I can't sort this out? Whose fault is it? Take some time to listen to this inner dialogue.

- Next, scan your body (you might need to start by noticing that you have one!). What are you experiencing? Sensations? Anywhere specifically? Heaviness? Tightness? Tension? Pressure? Hot or cold?

- Now, scan your thoughts. What are you thinking now after suggesting this dialogue to yourself? See if you can label the type of thinking. Obsession? Worry? Fear? Anger? Frustration? Rumination?

- Take a moment to note the effects on your body, your mind, your mood.

- Next, pause and take a few deep breaths and distract yourself. Think about the most recent TV show or movie you saw in order to get into a more neutral state.

- After you have returned to baseline, think again about the situation you originally brought to mind. Now you are ready to reframe it by thinking of it as a challenge, an opportunity, a place to break new ground with new learning.

- Ask yourself: what are the resources, abilities, tools, and skills I already have? This brings to mind your resources and positions you in an empowering way.

- Next, think of the outcome you would like to create. If you don't have a specific outcome in mind, think about creating the "best possible outcome" without having to know exactly what that might be.

- Now, ask yourself, who can help me create this outcome? What are the external resources I can mobilize to get assistance? How can I embrace the learning/ changes/challenges that this situation presents? Take a moment to suggest to yourself that you *already have all of the inner resources that you need in order to access and mobilize the external help* to create whatever outcome you want.

- Finally, picture yourself on the other side of the situation, having successfully negotiated it, having learned whatever lessons or assembled any tools you needed to create the desired (or best possible) outcome. From this place, scan your body. What do you notice? What are the sensations? Take a moment to scan your thoughts and your mood. Are they different in this frame?

Most people report feeling empowered, lighter, freer, calmer, and more creative in the "outcome frame." Just thinking about a problem within this framework can have a profound impact on how we feel.

....

When RAGE Runs the Show

Very close to the brain-body's FEAR system is the RAGE system. Both FEAR and RAGE signal us to either take flight from or fight danger. But in the case of RAGE, what began as a way to defend and protect has become a complicated mess that not only impacts our capacity to experience pleasure but gets in the way of good, satisfying sex. Many people find themselves in a nasty cycle: they develop a propensity for anger —

from angry moods to angry relationships. When RAGE and anger go untampered, frustration rules the day — especially when it comes to sex.

A case in point is Kara, a client whose perpetual anger has imploded her erotic life. Kara runs in for a session on her lunch break, in a rush as usual. And she is pissed off, also as usual. Some "stupid idiot" cut her off on the drive over. Kara is a recovering alcoholic in her late thirties, a single mother who works as a nurse in a nearby assisted living facility. Her current litany of complaints includes: her ex-husband is always late with the child support, her supervisor doesn't back her up when the families of problematic facility residents make unreasonable demands, and her fifteen-year-old son just got diagnosed with bipolar disorder. Kara isn't having any fun. And she isn't having any sex. Her fiancé, a mortgage broker and a "good guy," as she puts it, is fed up with her being irritable and angry. But what truly gets him is her total lack of sexual desire. She is never in the mood, and he's had it. This is the burning reason she is seeking treatment.

Kara's emotional basement is chock-full of trauma. She grew up in an unstable home. Her mom was a depressed alcoholic, in and out of treatment, and she never met her biological father. She and her mom moved frequently, usually because her mom was pursuing a new boyfriend. Two of her stand-in stepfathers were less than fatherly. She describes them as "baby men" who saw her as a burden and as a rival for her mom's attention.

I can see that despite this rough background, Kara is a tough cookie who has not at all given up on herself or on her desire for a "normal, happy life." She married early — twice, in fact — and she describes both of these previous relationships as "disasters" full of chaos, drama, and disappointment.

So, it makes perfect sense to me that Kara is angry — angry at her mother, her "faux" fathers, and probably herself. Indeed, Kara has had good reasons to be angry, and that anger most likely helped her survive the rough road she has traveled. But now the general baseline of her RAGE system is set at a high simmer, ready for a rolling boil. It's taking a toll on her relationships, her work, her sex life, and her connection with her kids. And it's also taking a toll on her health: she has recently been diagnosed with hypertension and prediabetes. Though it got her to seek therapy, her sexless relationship is only the tip of the iceberg. Her defensive emotional system needs to be harnessed and directed toward allowing her to experience any kind of healthy pleasure — and all kinds of healthy pleasure — for the sake of her overall health.

While some people might respond to this ongoing stress with fear or panic, it's Kara's personality to fight. She doesn't feel fear, only anger, and she directs a lot of this rage toward people who are supposed to be caretakers. Consciously, she knows her history predisposes her to being pissed off and chronically disappointed in others, as well as not trusting. But curiously, she also habitually sees herself as a victim of others.

What I immediately pick up on after hearing Kara's history and observing her behavior is that there seems to be a big disconnect between her knowing that she needs to change and actually being able to do so. For her to calm down her anger enough to be sexual, she needs first to listen to what is under the anger. The first step is to see how her anger began with a purpose. In her case, it served as an armor that protected her when she was a child and no one was appropriately taking care of her needs. Getting angry both warded off potential advances from a revolving queue of questionable "stepdads" and also enabled her to proclaim her needs, on the rare occasions someone was actually listening. But now, this anger habit is no longer serving her. Up until this point, it's been easier and safer for her to feel anger and present the defensive attitude of "I am going to fuck you before you fuck me." In fact, it's entrapping her. She needs to update her emotional responses so that they work for her in the here and now. Like many people stuck in RAGE, Kara is conflating being angry with feeling victimized. Somewhere along the way, Kara learned that she needed to make someone wrong in order to feel justified or entitled to feel angry.

Many people who have never had their feelings validated or accepted by caregivers have not internalized their own ability to self-validate. For most of her life, the only way Kara felt validated in her anger was when she could assign blame, which also enabled her to feel justified as a victim. One thing Kara needs to do in order to get out of her RAGE cycle is to consciously learn that she is entitled to feel whatever it is she feels, even if the cause isn't obvious or doesn't make sense — that this is a basic human right. But for Kara, like many people struggling to let go of this internal vision of herself as a victim, she does not believe that she is *intrinsically* deserving, worthy, and entitled — as she would have learned had the parenting she'd received been more consistent and attuned. Her early experiences of being a victim of inadequate parenting set up a pattern such that the only time she feels entitled to taking a stand for herself is when she feels wronged by others. Had Kara's feelings been both heard and validated by a consistent caretaker, not only would she have grown up to feel more deserving, she would have likely developed more skills in identifying and satisfying her own and others' emotional needs in a relationship (see "Good Sex Tool: Active Listening," part 2 validation exercise, page 147).

As her therapist, the challenge is to help her feel safe with me, so that she can truly experience and feel what underlies the rage, which I surmise to be fear.

How do I know that Kara is afraid?

Because as pissed off as she is about her boyfriend insisting she come in for treatment to get "fixed," she tells me that she needs to figure out what's going on "in the bedroom" because she is "afraid" that she is going to lose her boyfriend. In the past when she has come to this point in a relationship, where she withdraws from sex and intimacy, she typically sabotages the bond, letting her anger crash and burn it. What's different now is that at some level she has become aware of her own patterns: she has gained more insight into how she keeps repeating them over and over, and it is getting a bit stale. This is somewhat common as people get older — we become more aware of the negative consequences of our old strategies for deflecting or avoiding the real emotional issues. So as Kara has matured, she feels less ready to run and more motivated to understand herself.

And lucky for Kara, her fiancé is encouraging her to take time and energy to explore herself. He wants to make their relationship work. He even volunteered to come to sessions with her. He understands that they both need to learn and grow for the best possible outcome of their partnership. Reflecting more on his caring helps Kara shift the frame of therapy from fixing herself so she can provide sex for her partner to receiving love and support from her partner. In this way, Kara is recruiting her SEEKING and CARE systems to help balance her rage response. Instead of simply giving him what he wants (which would reinforce her rage and resentment), she begins to choose to accept his love and becomes happier, more playful, and generally more positive — and most importantly, less angry. The therapy and in particular the warm, fuzzy, and caring therapeutic connection she is forging with me, coupled with her enhanced understanding of the imbalanced defenses in her core emotions, has enabled her to feel safe and relaxed enough to bypass her anger and her fear and update her present feelings and desires.

Ultimately, in order to sustain these positive, affiliative emotions, Kara needs to heighten her SEEKING system and get more turned on by her life. She also has to let the love and support she receives in her relationship help heal her CARE system, so she can become more trusting of all of her relationships. (Since her relationship with her mother and then with most of her partners and ex-husbands were transactional, she operated on the premise of giving to get, just trying to meet her most basic needs.) Now she is focused on receiving. My attention, her attention, and her willingness to finally express her vulnerability is truly her power. Indeed, true acceptance of oneself allows for the power of transparency and vulnerability, which will replenish her natural desire to be sexual with her fiancé.

All of us have this built-in capacity for affiliative emotions, including LUST. In Kara's case, she needed to relax and feel safe in order to get out of defense mode. A few weeks into therapy, I ask Kara "What do you really want, Kara? Do you want to have sex?" And her response is an unequivocal "Yes!" The natural flow of her LUST emerges! As you can see from Kara's story, she came in fiery and pissed off and she left much more soft and open. How does RAGE take over so dramatically? Of all the seven systems, RAGE is the most conceptually complex.

Dismantling RAGE

In the most basic way, RAGE, like FEAR, operates primarily as a built-in defense system. Indeed, in experiments, this circuit "lights up" with electrical stimulation of the brain. Studies have also shown that this underlying neurobiological structure is further articulated and reinforced by specific neurochemicals. The RAGE system acts in response to glutaminergic and cholinergic recruitment, especially as the anger becomes more defensive in nature. However, there are major inhibitory neurochemicals that are designed to calm down this system, including the various brain opioid systems, GABA, and serotonin.

Let's unpack this neurobiology further. The hypothalamus, which we mentioned briefly earlier (chapter 3), is a key player here. It is a structure deep within the brain responsible for controlling many behaviors, including eating, drinking, temperature regulation, and sexual motivation. The hypothalamus also serves as the boss of the autonomic nervous system (ANS) and influences hormones through control of the master gland, the pituitary. In case you are a bit rusty on the nervous system, the ANS controls smooth muscle, like the tissues in your stomach and blood vessels, plus the glands, heart, and other internal organs. The ANS has two divisions — the sympathetic component, which, simply put, mobilizes the body in responses such as flight or fight, and the parasympathetic component, which is typically conceptualized as the body's chill-out system — responsible for storing and restoring energy.

If you are like most, you are not a big fan of being enRAGED. And that's probably a good thing since, as Panksepp noted, RAGE tends to backfire if not properly harnessed. At the very least RAGE triggers defenses in others, which tends to be self-defeating. At its worst, RAGE is the source of emotional hijacking, with potentially dire consequences. The usual scenario is one we have already described: when a lover or spouse finds a partner fornicating with someone else. And yes, this could be viewed as a limbic hijacking of the RAGE system. Sexual jealousies are rooted somewhere in the mammalian brain basement. In fact, one of the surest ways of eliciting RAGE activation in the male mammal nested with a female sexual partner is to introduce another male into the mix. Some aspects of RAGE reactivity appear to be genetically inherited, as has been supported by studies showing the heritability of aggression. And we do know that the tendency toward RAGE is fostered in children who are abused, sensitized by early experiences, and primed to flare. There are individual differences in the tonality of all emotional wired-in systems, including RAGE, an intersection of genetics (what nature has given us), and environmental factors/learning (nurture).

We want to remember that we have the opportunity to regulate our emotions using the advanced skills that can be honed via our higher brain centers, especially as we develop more insight and understanding of how the emotional basement and midlevel minds work. Top-down thinking can either inflame or soothe RAGE; the difference becomes a matter of how well a person can harness his or her parasympathetic system (the calming system). RAGE can be redirected constructively, or it can explode destructively.

For example: Imagine that you're driving home alone after a rather grueling day at the office. As you navigate the rush hour traffic, you contemplate the events of your day, and begin ruminating about how unfair it was that a coworker took credit for the success of a project that was originally your baby. You notice a car ahead of you weaving aggressively between lanes. Now on alert, you feel a tinge of adrenaline as you watch this "jerk" maneuver in front of you, and try to keep your distance. Your heart is already racing, fueled by irritation at the misbehaving coworker and the driver who thinks he is Mario Andretti competing at the Daytona 500. Lost for a minute in reverie, you notice that the cars ahead of you are stopping, and the daredevil driver cuts into your lane abruptly, causing you to hit the brake hard in order not to rear-end him. You manage to stop just short of his bumper. You feel your heart galloping, your blood boiling, and you are full-tilt furious. This is the perfect recipe for road rage.

Let's take another look at the same scenario. You are driving home from work with a trusted confidante who knows that you are peeved by the coworker who took credit for your pet project. Your friend agrees that it was indeed unfair, but reassures you that you will eventually get the credit you deserve once the dust settles. You realize that your friend is probably right, and you remind yourself that your boss isn't dumb; he knows how valuable you are to all projects. You and your friend acknowledge that the credit-seeking coworker is young and inexperienced. You decide to have a chat with him tomorrow — give the kid the benefit of the doubt — but at the same time set him straight.

Your attention returns to navigating the traffic, which is becoming increasingly congested. Out of the corner of your eye, you see an aggressive driver weaving from lane to lane. So does your passenger. You keep an eye on the wild driver. As you continue on, your friend mentions that most drivers these days seem to be in a terrible rush to go nowhere. You agree. When the driver swerves ahead of you, you see him, anticipating the cars slowing ahead, and react, applying the brakes forcefully but in enough time to stop gracefully. Your heart is beating fast in response to the situation. You take a deep breath and feel grateful that you dodged this bullet. Sure, this driver's behavior is reckless and stupid, but there's no need to let it boil your blood. What's the point, you think? Maybe the guy has a problem. Your friend reaches out to touch your arm, noting your skillful driving. You both sigh in relief, and then continue on home.

As Panksepp and others have noted, the ability to constructively and productively express anger (what is cognitively layered over the RAGE system) is key to emotional balance. Neither RAGING with anger nor bottling it up is healthy for an individual or his/her relationships. With cultivated self-awareness you can employ your higher-level brain to help you make the necessary shifts so that neither fear nor anger will block your path to pleasure. If you think you are prone to an inner voice saying, "Danger, Will Robinson, danger," you may just have an overactive fear response. If you are often withdrawing from social occasions or work challenges for fear of rejection, this may be the case as well. On the other hand, you might find yourself raging like Kara, always on the defense, waiting for a fight or to be taken advantage of. Regardless, these fear and rage responses are often cognitive distortions that "ooze up" from the midlevel mind, where they are embedded memories that are no longer even accurate and, if left to fester, will indeed rob you of pleasure.

....

Good Sex Tool: Unpacking Anger

Whether big or small, unpacking RAGE begins with recognizing that you are in RAGE mode. Then, you can defuse this
emotion so it doesn't take over. Try this quick exercise in somatic breathing that will bring your body into a calm state.

1. Sit in a comfortable position.

2. Close your eyes.

3. Breathe in through your nostrils.

4. Breathe out through your mouth, extending your out
   breath, and focus on releasing the sensations in your
   body to the gentle pull of gravity.

5. Check in with yourself: how are you feeling?

6. If you still feel angry, then walk, jump, or engage in
   some other mild exercise to further release the pent-up
   adrenaline.

....

It's important to keep in mind that our defenses originate as nonconscious and automatic — both anger and fear were originally meant
to be mechanisms of protection. However, as we've evolved into more
complex beings, and as the original biological imperative has taken on
psycho-social layering, our defenses often just get in our way. Indeed,
these defensive responses can trigger one another and exacerbate additional emotional imbalances. The result? A cascade effect of nonhelp-
ful responses that further erode our relationships and our capacity for
pleasure. Katie was suffering from an outdated FEAR response and Kara
was suffering from RAGE that was getting in the way of PLAY, CARE,

and LUST. Again, these basic core emotions are powerful forces that live within us and our memories. Unless we notice them and connect to how they are playing out or emerging in our thoughts, feelings, behaviors, and body responses, they will continue to interfere with our access to and experience of our pleasure system. And, when it comes to FEAR and RAGE, these defensive emotions can easily wreak havoc on all aspects of our lives.

In order to come into better balance, we can use our SEEKING system to improve CARE, PLAY, and LUST, so that we can ultimately access the pleasure we so desire. Fortunately, we are all inherently flexible and can learn new ways of relating to ourselves and others that tamp down our defensive emotions and pump up our affiliative emotions, those that are PLAYful and LUSTful and enable us to feel an exuberance for life.

6

CARE, GRIEF, and PLAY:
Using Our Affiliative Emotions
to Enhance Pleasure

I t goes without saying that without CARE — the love, bonding, and security that comes with companionship — human beings can't survive. We are without a doubt wired to seek out and receive caring attachments. How does the brain ensure this need gets met? It has a built-in CARE system that drives parents (usually the mother) to care for the offspring, which will happen automatically in nonhuman animals; in people these built-in "maternal feelings" can be viewed more as an evolutionarily instilled predisposition to care for babies rather than a hardwired instinct. And as mentioned, in the brain, this CARE system works in concert with the PANIC/GRIEF system, creating a network of functions that lead directly to our pleasure pathway. It's the job of the PANIC/GRIEF system to remind us of our need for CARE. It's also a reminder that we are not meant to be isolated or live alone. We are made to live in the context of a family group, tribe, or larger network of community systems.

But like all the other systems, this pair can also become unbalanced — with either too much CARE or too little, triggering hypervigilance in the PANIC/GRIEF system. And sometimes even in the case where parenting has been more than adequate, some people, as Lady Gaga would say, are just born this way. We saw this clearly in Tim's case: he was born with nervous wiring.

Whatever the cause, if someone becomes overwrought, they live in a constant state of high anxiety or experience panic attacks. People who have experienced early trauma that involves loss of a caregiver (through separation or lack of availability) often show this high degree of PANIC/GRIEF, leaving them anxious, fearful, and unable to connect. On the other side of the spectrum, overparenting, where the caregiver, responding to his or her own issues, is not attuned to what the child actually needs, can also wreak havoc with the tonality of the child's PANIC/GRIEF *and* CARE systems. As we will see, in general, imbalances in the CARE system can contribute to shutting down SEEKING and in its wake, LUST. Let's take a look at how these two systems must work in tandem to be optimally balanced for pleasure.

Early Attachments as Foundation for CARE System

Early childhood experiences fundamentally shape the basic tonality of both the CARE and the PANIC/GRIEF systems. While there may indeed be genetic predispositions that affect the reactivity of these systems to begin with, the quality of our earliest social bonds with primary caretakers essentially forms the basis for how securely we view ourselves in the world, either dialing up the anxious style or dialing down the wired-in reactivity. Having our earliest needs met with attunement, warmth, and reliability, we grow into feeling that our needs are okay and that people will be generally happy to help us get them met. This is what psychologists refer to as secure attachment.

If, however, early attachment is severely lacking or inconsistent, two main forms of insecure attachment can develop. Attachment styles are laid down by early experiences in concert with your inherited temperament (which refers to how reactive your defensive systems are by nature). The wired-in bottom brain is influenced by ongoing midlevel mind's classical conditioning, which is why our early childhood emotional experiences are so powerful in affecting lifelong tonality of the seven core systems.

When it comes to attachment, there are two main flavors of insecure attachment and both stem from disruptions in the defensive systems — one in the FEAR system, one in the PANIC/GRIEF system — and they both affect how we relate to others, especially in romantic relationships:

(1) Anxious or preoccupied attachment shows up as, "my relationships aren't safe and secure." "I need my connections to be okay in order for me to be okay." Such a setup often means that women and men will choose the needs of the relationship or partner over the self — a style that results in a person not standing up for their own needs. Learning how to voice your own needs is an important feature of healthy relationships. On the contrary, developing habits for relationship success involves learning that not taking a stand for ourselves is as much of a relationship offense and often, over the long run, as destructive as the more dramatic offenses of lying and cheating.

(2) Avoidant — don't choose a relationship at all. Can look like "I am not good enough for others," which keeps people from forming relationships at all. Or alternatively, "others aren't good enough for me" — the dismissive type of avoidant anxiety that leads to the person creating

a trail of superficial relationships with others who are
left behind because of not measuring up to ridiculous
standards or unrealistic expectations. Often the dismissive type of individual shows up as a person with major
commitment issues.

Understanding your attachment style and the tonality of your
wired-in defensive systems can free you from the negative ramifications
of what amounts to a perpetual altered state of alarm and harness that
energy through top-down messages that foster rebalancing the bottom
brain systems. (If you are curious to learn more about your own attachment style, you can find many questionnaires online; you can also find
more information in the endnotes. This information about yourself and
others can also help you gain insight into how you form and nurture relationships.)

At a neurobiological level, both the giving and the receiving of care
is activated by internal opioids — our brains' own endogenous (internally produced) pleasure pumpers and painkillers. These neurochemicals make sure that we attach — to our young, our mates, our parents,
and friends — and are released automatically when women give birth
so they attach to their young, are released during sex, and are even released during caring conversations. One of the central neurochemicals
activated by touch is oxytocin.

In order to foster nurturance, mothers release the hormone oxytocin
— facilitating tenderness on the one hand, and strong protective impulses toward our young on the other. And when infants do not receive
sufficient CARE, they die. But oxytocin is not just released by mothers
after childbirth. Oxytocin is liberally released with touch (and also with
sexual behavior and orgasm, as my own studies have indicated). Don't
believe, however, all of what you read in the media about oxytocin as the

"cuddle or love" hormone. The media tends to oversimplify. The way oxytocin works is way more complicated.

It's more accurate to suggest that oxytocin's effects are context dependent and seem to be more related to the molecule's antianxiety effects (potentially in concert with oxytocin-facilitated opioid activity), thereby acting as a stress reducer during our interpersonal encounters, whether it be during simple conversation or through reassuring physical touch. In other words, oxytocin release seems to have at least two general purposes: to make us feel good and to be good for us. When I teach physiological psychology, I amuse my students by calling dopamine the "slutty neurotransmitter" in that it gets released with nearly every kind of feel-good drug or experience. And dopamine appears to have a very close and personal relationship with oxytocin, sharing a positive interaction in which they tend to boost each other's functions, so much so that researchers are considering that disturbances in the oxytocin/dopamine dance may underlie some serious mental health issues. And conversely, finding a way to enhance the dopamine/oxytocin relationship may have some awesome clinical applications in the treatment of mood and social-affiliative disorders as well as addiction. One low-tech way to dial up this dopamine dance is to engage in lots of caring touch and playful sex. In short, we need real face-to-face, eye-to-eye, flesh-to-flesh communion with our "conspecifics," which is a fancy way to say organisms of our own species. This is an urgent biological need — one that far too many are going without, especially in this tech-driven culture that has created a digital divide among us.

Again, when the CARE system becomes dysregulated, we will be more vulnerable to feeling emotionally upset or have difficulty connecting to others. An inherited tendency toward emotional system imbalances in the basement of the brain (a biological factor) in concert with early childhood experiences that were not very caring (psychological/

learning) in the context of a culture that doesn't truly prioritize our face-to-face and flesh-to-flesh social bonds (social) is a recipe for disaster. This can result in reliance on external drugs, compulsive sex, or eating (or something else) to ease the psychological pain of absence of care. Indeed, this state triggers the PANIC/GRIEF system to backfire, creating yet even more pain.

The GRIEF component of the continuum also gets triggered when we lose a loved one. If it's out of balance, you might be so mired in depression that you avoid the connections that you so desperately need — resulting in perpetual sadness and loneliness. And conversely, if the PANIC component of the PANIC/GRIEF system is out of balance and overfunctioning, you might be hypersensitive to any threat to your connections — either real or imagined — prompting you to be clingy.

When aroused, GRIEF will naturally make us feel misery and distress. However, through time and healing and normal processing of a loss, we can revert back to safety of our CARING, secure relationships. When we are fortunate to be deeply embedded in social supports and surrounded by sources of CARE, we usually experience a feeling of well-being, which in turn strengthens the very social bonds that elicit it in a wonderful positive cycle of CARE, creating yet more CARE and comfort.

As you may have experienced, the undesired breakup of an important romantic relationship is often accompanied by signs of withdrawal — an aching longing for the beloved that actually feels like a pain in the heart. There can be ruminations; obsessive thoughts about what went wrong, furtive dreams of restoring the connection, followed by alterations to our appetites, our sleep patterns, agitation, depression, and even impaired immunity. Sounds a bit like recovering from an addiction, yes? For some, the breakup of a romantic relationship can be as incapacitating as withdrawing from drugs of abuse, especially for those whose emotional systems are out of balance to begin with.

Let's take a look at how this CARE-PANIC continuum can dampen LUST and PLAY in real life.

When Overactive CARE Dampens PLAY and LUST

Bill and Liza are a thirtysomething couple living in New York City with two kids in a small apartment that was meant to be temporary. They met while working together as midlevel managers at a small advertising firm. Liza decided to quit to be a stay-at-home mom so, with less income, the small apartment became less temporary and more confining.

Although Liza feels she's doing the right thing by staying home to take care of her two kids, both of whom are under two years of age, the marriage is suffering. It has been months since they've had sex, and when they have, it's been awful. Liza admittedly just goes through the motions, leaving Bill feeling slighted and depressed. Liza used to be fun. Big fun. And Bill was thrilled at having met a soulmate who seemed to be compatible in and out of the bedroom. But now, after a day with the kids climbing all over her, Liza doesn't feel like being touched, and doesn't have the slightest interest in sex. Her CARE system is overwrought, raising levels of both oxytocin and prolactin, which in turn downregulate (i.e., lower) estrogen and testosterone, dampening both her SEEKING system and LUST. And her husband's whining is not helping matters.

Up until now, Bill has been patient, but he is reaching his limit. He insists on how much he loves Liza and wants to give her space and room to figure things out. But he's frustrated. "I didn't get married to not have sex," Bill complains. He explains during a session that he has to literally beg for an occasional hand- or blowjob during which Liza looks dreadfully bored and uninspired.

Liza feels that Bill's anger is unfair. "We have the luxury of a weekly

babysitter on Friday nights, and after a drink or two I finally loosen up."
Bill chimes in, "She promises that she will get back her groove."

They kiss and fondle each other at the restaurant, but once they hit
the lobby of the apartment building, it's like a bucket of ice water gets
dumped on Liza's only slightly ignited lost libido. It is as if Liza's libido is
conditioned to turn off the minute she returns home.

What's going on with these two?

Liza is manifesting symptoms of an imbalance at the bottom of the
brain. You are in "tend and befriend/mothering brain," I tell her. I explain the seven systems and then say, "Your CARE system is cockblock-
ing your LUST system."

I also reassure her that this is very common for new parent couples.
"This happens to some people. And that's okay. If you understand how
you are wired at the bottom of the brain, you will understand why your
sexual energy feels out of reach right now. You used to experience spontaneous or active sexual desire when you were first together. But it's
really common for women, and some men, to lose some or all of their
spontaneous sexual desire.

"I mean, honestly, Liza," I explain, "if you factor in the 24-7 childcare
you are doing, it makes total sense that your erotic energy is turned way
down. Everything is actually working for the most part, but we need to
help you find your balance."

Liza's universe has shrunk and everything hinges on the babies. All
of her regular pleasurable activities take a back seat — friends, free time,
travel, going out — altering the dynamic of the wired-in systems. Her
stress that comes with the nonstop taking care of kids depletes her calls
for dopamine, so there is nothing to signal SEEKING, PLAY, or LUST.

As long as the CARE system stays overactivated, it will downregulate
the LUST system as well as the PLAY system. If not able to pursue regu-

lar pleasures, Liza's SEEKING system is hijacked and devoted to CARE. This situation is further reinforced by our society, which tends to value mothers who give up their time and energy for the sake of their children. If new parents are fortunate enough to have a good amount of social support, family members nearby ready and willing to give them frequent breaks from perpetual childcare, if their worlds are set up to encourage them to continue the playful and lustful pursuits of adults, they may be lucky enough to have the abundance of time and energy for self-nurture and partner pleasuring that could inoculate them from this loss of PLAY and LUST. That, however, is a lot of ifs, given the fevered pace of modern life and the mobility of the nuclear family frequently resulting in isolation from extended families who might be able to help.

Like many couples in similar positions, Bill and Liza need to come up with their own solution to their marriage and their almost nonexistent sex life. The plan for them begins counterintuitively — with Liza giving herself permission to NOT have sex in general. Then, with the pressure off and Liza free to find ways to get turned on by her life in general (and turning up the energy in her SEEKING system), she will naturally refind some passion beyond the full-time caretaking. The probable result? Liza will again discover her LUST for life . . . and for Bill. And Bill will no doubt be ready and appreciative of Liza's return.

I know that their therapy will not take much time. One critical lesson from the habits for relationship success is to acknowledge that we must view our partner's needs as being just as important as our own. As soon as Liza registers the need for her to truly commit to finding a solution that works for both of them, and then understands her own imbalance, she becomes more motivated to address this issue, not just to please her husband, but for her own good. In the long run, rebalancing her energies will help keep her relationship from stalling and keep her from collapsing into her role as a parent instead of staying a separate person and a partner. This process means that Liza and Bill truly learn to listen to each other and recognize and respect their respective needs. And for this, I direct them to an exercise called Active Listening (below). Once Liza begins to actively take care of herself, and she and Bill are more clear about how each of them feels, then the healing takes off.

She books a weekend at a yoga retreat for herself (alone!) to start her new yoga life, and also signs up for a weekly class at a local studio. Even though we agree that she gets "time off" from being expected to have sex so she can find a way to tap into her sensual appetite, I explain to Liza that sometimes desire can kick in after arousal is initiated — and that there are lots of ways to get aroused — this is what we call receptive desire. Liza decides she likes the sound of one of the exercises I learned from a sex therapist and sex educator, Dr. William Stayton, which involves getting a hard copy of the famous sex manual *The Joy of Sex* and encouraging the clients to invent games to play together. Liza takes the initiative to set up two weekly "playdates" with Bill during which they take turns randomly opening up pages of the book and then engaging in conversations about what they like or don't like about the particular sexual behaviors. Then they schedule sessions of active listening, going through the index of the book and challenge each other to talk about the particular subjects, taking risks to share whatever comes to mind, to explore their own separate sexual fantasies, experiences, turn-ons and turn-offs, reaching in to penetrate each other's inner worlds. And of course, since they are "prohibited" from actually having sex, this exercise feels safe and playful to Liza. Almost predictably, the "idea" that they aren't supposed to have sex makes it all feel new and exciting.

Liza reports back that she is getting increasingly interested in having sex with Bill now that she sees him with "new eyes." They surprise themselves by learning that there is a lot that they still don't know about themselves and each other. These new sex conversations have opened up many more honest, probing, interesting explorations of their lives in general. Bill rings a few weeks later to say that Liza decided, herself, to break the "no sex" rule and give Bill a very enthusiastic blowjob after a particularly hot playdate. It would appear that Liza has managed to get back her groove.

....

Good Sex Tool: Active Listening, part 1

As individual clients dig into their emotional basement, I try to get them to connect outside of themselves as well. One tool that works well to begin the thread of communication between partners who have lost connection (for whatever reason) is called Active Listening, which asks couples to set aside time where you and your partner truly listen and actually hear each other, one at a time. In fact, I often suggest that couples "give each other sessions" so they can air all their thoughts, feelings, frustrations, fears, and doubts in a safe space. The partner's job is to listen—not judge or try to fix or defend themselves. The listener tries to repeat exactly what the speaker says—to get each and every word, idea, thought, and feeling expressed treated as precious jewels to be heard and appreciated. As the talking and listening occur, the person speaking experiences a peak and release of the feelings and then a letting go of the resentments.

These sessions work best when you have decided ahead of time on the duration, and I always recommend starting slowly. Try it for ten minutes and then gradually, with practice, extend it to about thirty minutes. As I tell my clients, if you can learn to tolerate your feelings about your partner's thoughts and feelings, you can hold a magnificent space for personal and relationship transformation.

Directions for basic Active Listening:

1. Establish that both of you are in the right frame of mind to do the session and decide who will be the speaker and who will be the active listener.

2. Make a clear agreement that you are doing a session and that what is said in the session stays in the session (what happens in Vegas stays in Vegas).

3. Set the timer.

4. The speaker starts talking and tries to keep the sound bites short enough so the listener can take it all in.

5. The listener repeats back what he/she has heard. For example, "What I hear you saying is . . ." Upon completion, the listener then asks, "Is that correct?"

6. The speaker indicates yes or no, and if the listener missed something or did not hear the speaker's meaning accurately, then the speaker repeats the information. The listener then repeats the corrected information.

7. The listener then asks, "Is there anything more you'd like to add?"

The point is to stick to the precise information the speaker is sharing without adding your own interpretations, angles, attempts to influence, fix, or otherwise embellish what your partner is actually saying. Keep it simple. Sticking to the script creates the safe space to communicate within the exercise and interrupts the usual habits of conversation.

....

Soothing PANIC/GRIEF Imbalances and Finding a Whole New You

Janet is a forty-nine-year-old, attractive, Ivy-League educated woman. Despite a ton of money in the bank, having had a successful career as a doctor, and being able to retire ridiculously early to follow her "bliss," she is unable to summon passion for the next leg of her journey, or a partner to share it. She is always, always anxious — a definite tip-off that her GRIEF/PANIC system is in overdrive.

Janet originally came to see me because of the pain she experienced after a difficult breakup. She has been married twice. She ended the first one when it became clear to her that her husband was chronically angry, miserable in all areas of his life, and he wouldn't go to therapy. She got tired of dealing with his temper tantrums and harsh criticism, so she moved on. A second marriage a few years later seemed promising. This husband was gentler, more fun, and more functional overall. But Janet was devastated when she learned that he was having an affair with an old girlfriend who had dumped him years before. She wanted to save the marriage, but when he chose instead to leave Janet for the other woman, she had no choice.

Since the second divorce, Janet has become isolated and withdrawn, unable to date or even spark interest in online dating sites. She used to think this was because her job as an ER doctor was too stressful. But now, after retiring, she still has trouble sleeping, still can't lose the twenty

pounds she's gained, and ruminates endlessly about what she isn't doing with her life. She doesn't like her body enough to be open to dating
anyone new since she got divorced. She worries that any boyfriend will
only want her for her money, so spends a lot of time at home, looking
at Facebook, feeling lonely and blue. And she is feeling worse than ever
because she thought she would feel better once she quit work. Indeed,
she has made a lot of money and also inherited additional wealth. But all
the years of not being taken care of by her parents emotionally have left
her with a feeling of scarcity and difficulty taking care of herself. All the
money in the bank and she can't spend a dime on herself.

In our work together, we have been exploring the skeletons in her
emotional basement, paying particular attention to the depletion in her
CARE system due to the emotional neglect of her parents and their reliance on her to take care of them, especially her mother. In my opinion,
she is spending way too much time alone and when she does hang out
with friends, she always seems to be doing for them, not simply being
with them. Friends know that Janet has money, so they turn to her when
in need. She is the one who fields phone calls from ailing aunts and troubled cousins when a medical issue arises and they want free advice. Even
ex-lovers turn to Janet with requests for consults when family members'
health fails. There's a lot of give and not a lot of get for Janet, so her social
interactions cannot do much to feed her CARE or PLAY systems.

In addition, her lack of appetite for anything to nurture herself—
work, social engagements, intellectual pursuits, and dating—all point
to a depressed (downregulated) SEEKING system. When I trace back
the CARE-PANIC/GRIEF disequilibrium to her formative attachments
with her parents, I discover that her parents, now deceased, were both
survivors of the Holocaust.

Janet's parents were too preoccupied with their own issues to pay
good attention to her. This is not to blame her parents.

As we get to know one another, Janet tells me that her mother was so needy that all of her father's energy focused on her mother, with nothing left for young Janet. As an adult, this stunted CARE system resulted, in part, in a long line of taking care of broken guys — even the last husband who she thought was going to take care of her. She never felt totally comfortable with others socially, and always felt like something was essentially wrong with her. To cope with this discomfort, she focused on taking care of others, which made her feel worthy and wanted — with and through being needed. But by focusing her energies on taking care of others, Janet never focused appropriately on making sure her own needs were taken care of, mostly because she didn't feel entitled to even meet her own needs. This is important information for me to understand and explains why Janet's parents are very much still present to her in a loop of automatic, emotionally infused negative self-talk that continues to condition her to be afraid, to not trust, and to think she is not "good enough" to dare to be happy. These thoughts are so ubiquitous that she experiences them as the wallpaper of her mind.

Janet's anxiety, depleted CARE system, and overactive PANIC/ GRIEF system are clearly overwhelming her. She's done therapy before — with some benefit. It actually helped her get out of the first marriage gone bad and to cope with the challenges of her former medical career, but now she is looking to really and truly get out of her own way and needs help knowing how to start.

Because of the inherited trauma from her parents' experience, it's clear that we needed to dig a lot deeper into Janet's bio/psycho/social networking to understand and parse out what is at the heart of the imbalanced CARE-PANIC system.

In order to make her feel more whole, her therapy needs to pump up her social engagement system such that she can learn how to take risks and ask people for what she needs and wants. We engage her SEEKING system so that she can become more curious than afraid. Indeed, her parents, who were so socially withdrawn, squashed her natural social curiosity and reinforced her awkwardness. Once her relationships become more stable, with and through the increasing comfort with her own needs, then she can feel safe enough to explore all of her feelings. I suggest two specific ways for her to initiate this: to branch out and create a new network of close friends and to stoke her SEEKING system through play, curiosity, and other interests.

Janet essentially begins to work on developing a repaired secure attachment style that modifies her inner soundtrack to sound more like "I am okay and the world is okay, too." This process is all about helping her put attention on how she can develop the fine art of self-care, which for Janet and so many people like her, requires learning new boundaries with the people in her life. She has to learn to say no to invitations or requests that are set up to position her in the habitual caretaker role. She needs to discern more carefully who to let into her life. This new learning takes time. But the good news is now that Janet understands the imbalances in her emotional basement — the overactive PANIC/GRIEF and underactive self-CARE systems — she can use this awareness to give herself choices and direction. Using hypnotherapy suggestions in sessions, we ground a new belief system that helps her embrace the tools and resources within herself to create everything she needs and wants in her life (see Accessing Your Inner Resources exercise, below). She gets to say yes to herself. She gets to tell others that it doesn't work for her to always respond to their needs and requests. She gets to make space for play and exploration of her own needs and passions.

The CARE-GRIEF continuum will always impact the tonality of the other systems. Understanding how these systems may or may not be in balance, overactive or underactive, will help you gain insight into your relationship dynamics, as well as your capacity to seek out pleasure in and of itself. As we will see with Janet, once she starts to re-balance her PANIC/GRIEF system with more CARE, her PLAY and LUST systems will get rekindled. Indeed, PLAY is a huge factor in ultimately resuscitating LUST and SEEKING, bringing balance to both these core systems.

....

Good Sex Tool: Accessing Your Inner Resources

An important tenet of my work with women and men who are trying to get out from under their emotional baggage is to remind them that they have all the internal resources to create what they want externally in their lives. This idea is directly adapted from Ericksonian hypnotherapy, which is my go-to method. However, you don't need to do hypnotherapy on yourself in order for this exercise to work for you. The most important part of this inner resource work is to suggest to yourself that you indeed *already have all of the internal resources that you need to have all of the external resources you need and want.* **This creates a sense of relaxation and safety that makes us even more resourceful.**

1. Find yourself a quiet space where you will not be disturbed. Feel free to drop into your breath. Keep it simple — take a long smooth inhalation and then a longer smooth exhalation.

2. Begin by giving yourself full permission to be exactly as you are in this moment. And then, give this moment full permission to be exactly as it is. The way to access your

inner resources is to start where you are. *Full permission to simply be as you are.*

3. Then allow yourself to go just a little bit deeper into the realization that you have an incredible abundance of resources that can be accessed with positive suggestion.

4. Remind yourself that *your mind is very creative.* Put that creativity in motion by asking yourself, *"I wonder how I can access the inner tools, skills, insights, abilities, possibilities, and resources I need to create what I want and need in my life?"* When we ask a question in this way, embedded in the phrase *"I wonder how I can?"* is the statement *"I can!"*

As mentioned, our minds can organically come up with amazing insights, options, and solutions with no effort at all. In fact, sometimes thinking too much at the top of the mind just gets in the way of intuitive problem solving. And remember, the best part of accessing your inner resources and having your needs met is that you don't have to do this alone. You already have all of the inner resources to create all the people, places, and circumstances that you'll ever need to meet your external needs and access your external resources.

As we drop in to the realization that we can indeed access external resources through mobilizing our inner resources, we can loosen and soften attachment to things looking a certain way in any moment—whether it be outcomes with particular people or circumstances. Basically, the less anxious we become about specific outcomes, the more relaxed, resourceful and resilient, and creative we can be. How does this play out? We become able to recognize that if one love relationship is not going to last in spite of our best intentions and efforts, then we will eventually find satisfaction and partnership elsewhere. If our dream job doesn't pan out, we trust that there are many other possibilities that may actually provide enhanced opportunities in the long run. If a friend disappoints us, we can take it less personally and look for support from those who are truly available. This reframing dials down our anxiety about needing something or someone to be a certain way and permits us to be more present and appreciative of what is, which becomes a recipe for cultivating a secure attachment style in which we feel that our needs are okay and that the world will generally help us meet them.

Using this practice is like going to the mind/emotion resources gym. When we intentionally remind ourselves that we do indeed have access to everything we need or want through our own resourcefulness, our connection to our own inner resources is strengthened, like a muscle that gets used. We can flex and strengthen our superpowers of SEEKING, self-CARE, CARE for others, and PLAY.

....

The Wondrous Potential of PLAY

Henry is a fit and attractive fifty-eight-year-old married man who is a partner in a big litigation law firm. He has a type A personality and has gotten far in his life because of his hard work, resilience, and tendency toward perfectionism. He loves his work and cares deeply about his wife of thirty years as well as everyone he loves. On the surface, Henry has it made — he has a great family and friends, does lots of charity work, takes plenty of trips, and has a beautiful home. But lately, Henry has been having some trouble with an area that has never given him trouble before. The erections that used to happen reliably aren't so reliable, and now he has begun avoiding sex with his wife, Lilly, due to embarrassment. He hasn't tried Viagra yet since he thinks that is "cheating."

"My penis should work on its own like it always has," he asserts. "I have been checked out by my family doctor, a cardiologist, and a urologist, and they tell me that everything seems to be fine."

I talk with Henry a bit about his history and find out that his dad died at age sixty of a heart attack after a long struggle with coronary heart disease. I ask him how this event affected him; he says he doesn't really worry about it. "I am in terrific health, have been seeing a cardiologist proactively, exercise regularly, and generally do everything that I am supposed to so my heart health is that of a much younger man, my doctors assure me."

So, Henry's body doesn't seem to be the issue here. It is his head. He is suffering from a bad case of "spectatoring," the condition where self-consciousness and performance anxiety shut down the sexual response. Once he had had erectile issues (which happen to all men at some point) with his wife on a number of occasions, his head took over and he was unable to be present and in the moment enough to allow the sexuality to unfold.

So what's happening with Henry and his penis?

When I ask what comes to mind when he thinks about fear, his eyes widen, suddenly figuring it out. He says, "Now that I think about it . . . My father died at the age that I am now. I guess I'm afraid that I will die like him."

We dig a bit further into his childhood. He was sent to boarding school and expected to "grow up quick." He explains, "I remember feeling like I always had to be a man, not a kid."

For all of its great potential, the impulse to play is actually quite fragile and can be easily overridden if we feel stressed or unsafe. Henry seems to have skipped over play and now, fifty-odd years later, his PANIC/GRIEF system is too panicky. It makes sense given what we know about Henry's history. His dad's protracted illness, the looming threat of loss, the derailment of his childhood have all taken their toll on his capacity to relax into sex. As his PANIC system engages, the physiological state of relaxation conducive to sexual arousal is not easily accessible.

I explain to Henry that as men age, penises aren't always as cooperative as they used to be. It makes sense that his capacity for lasting erections may simply be slightly diminished. But Henry is so goal oriented — "focused on getting the job done" — that he is forgetting to be present to his experience, and this is also taking a toll. I suggest that he learn to increase the play factor in his life. And he needs to tamp down his impulse to care so much for others — a way of thinking that puts him in the mode of the overly conscientious, seriously successful master of the universe. Of course, I don't want to undermine the fact that he wants to take CARE of his wife, but I do want him to want to loosen up a bit.

Our therapy then focuses on fostering a sense of PLAY in approaching sexuality. We map out specific suggestions that he can use to turn up the PLAY and LUST systems. I tell him to imagine himself on the other side of this challenge — where he is effortlessly enjoying an outrageously satisfying sex life with his wife — one that delights them both.

He begins to see his future self as a present, feeling, playful explorer. Henry has pretty quickly figured out that he can get past his worries if he simply lets himself feel his feelings — they will peak and release. Overactivated PANIC/GRIEF systems can be quelled by mindful discharge of the distress — whether it be by "taking a session" (see Active Listening exercises) to unpack the fears by sharing them with a partner or peer, or even by writing about them in a journal. Much research supports the notion that actively expressing our emotions with others yields great physical and emotional benefits — even decreasing inflammation which may be at the core of many illnesses.

What was important for Henry was acknowledging both his fear that he would have similar health issues to his dad and the pressure he has felt since he was a kid to "be a man." In being present with these fears and reinforcing the understanding that erectile issues are very normal for men of his age, Henry's anxiety can reduce and he can more easily play — in a sexual capacity, or otherwise.

He decides that he doesn't have to protect his wife from his anxieties, and once he opens up to her, they both feel more connected and close. He then puts his new plan into action by taking my suggestion to "play" with sensate focus exercises (see chapter nine) with his wife. These simple but powerful exercises developed by none other than Masters and Johnson involve the couple taking turns exploring each other's bodies (at first without touching the genitals or having any kind of sex). This is a powerful tool to help Henry find his way back to the moment, his wife, and to sensation and exploration rather than the kind of goal-directed focus that succeeds in the boardroom but doesn't work well in the bedroom.

In Henry's case, getting him to infuse his life with play helped to both balance out the overactive CARE system and quell the residual PANIC/GRIEF. I suggest that instead of all work and no play, Henry ease up on his volunteering and create time to relax and have fun — with his friends and his wife. With my coaching, Henry decides to do something he always fantasized about but would never previously have considered a worthwhile use of his time. He enrolls in an improv class at a local theater group and spends every Thursday evening learning how to be in the moment, how to listen intently, how to play with his peers while exploring new behavior. This kind of play actually flowed over into his sex life and enabled him to stop judging his not-as-reliable penis. Though the breath work and exploring the Bhandas (see Mula Bhandas exercise, page 150), Henry forged a deeper physical connection with his body, and in turn improved his erectile functioning, which of course boosted his LUST system and overall confidence

He rang me up a few weeks after our last session to say that he was having a blast goofing off in his spare time and had actually bought a Twister game to play with his wife. He said at first she thought he was nuts, but their game induced a bout of silly laughter in them that culminated in a roll in the hay. Henry was very pleased.

The bottom line is that play is good for your health. More play and more sex mean less stress and inflammation, and more protection from coronary heart disease (the disease that killed his dad).

A healthy working PLAY system is integral to a healthy and robust pleasure system. The PLAY system is literally the source of our social joy chemicals. Our ability to experience pleasure and its reverse state of anhedonia is closely tied to rebooting our body-brain connection so that we let ourselves PLAY. It sounds simple, and it is; but it's also a profound human experience and emotion that is necessary for our health and survival.

Now that we have an understanding of your seven baseline emotional systems, we can turn to the more dynamic aspects of emotional functioning. In the next couple of chapters, you get to try some additional tools and techniques that will both rebalance your core emotional systems and reboot your capacity for pleasure with a keen eye on finding your way to healthy hedonism — pleasures that feel good and are good for you. Get ready to roll!

Part Three

......

Pursuing—and Obtaining— Healthy Pleasures

7

Operational Intelligence and Creating a New Way to Be

One of the most important and helpful lessons I've learned is that happiness doesn't quite work like we think it does. In fact, we often have things pretty much backward. We think that if we do certain things, we will have what we want and need, and then we will be happy. For example, if I do something (go to grad school), I will have something (my PhD), and then I will be something (happy/satisfied/complete). Many of us convince ourselves that if we get the right relationship, the right job, the right house, the kids, the car, the hot tub — all of the possessions and accomplishments that we think we need and want — then, we will be happy.

Ahh.

But what actually ends up happening is that we suffer from what's known as the hedonic treadmill: we habituate to our new gains, and our happiness returns to our relative baselines fairly quickly. We each have a general set point of happiness (which is determined 50 percent by genetics, 10 percent by our circumstances, and 40 percent by the decisions we make and how we reinforce or adapt the genetic loading we are born with). The good news is that this set point can be modified or adjusted by consciously making decisions or choices — especially when it comes to managing our core emotional systems.

Another piece of good news is that the hedonic treadmill also works in reverse. We similarly adjust to negative events, even those that are really upsetting, and return to our relative set point of well-being. We humans are above all an adaptable species.

This emotional set point is made up of the interactions among any or all of our emotional core states. Understanding your set point goes a long way to understanding your general "way of being," that collection of habits that define your attitude, behaviors, reactions, and ways of inter-acting with others.

If 40 percent of our happiness resides in what we decide to do with the cards we are dealt, why not take advantage and harness the power of our attention, and deliberately and intentionally focus on how we get to be happy, satisfied, and complete right here and right now.

One overarching way to begin to create your new way to be is through the lens — and the tools — of what I call operational intelligence.

Operational Intelligence:
The Master/Mistress Is in the House

One fabulous realization about the inner workings of your brain is that you have more control over your life than you probably thought was pos-sible. But, as you've seen, we need to start with the bottom of the brain and work our way up to the more complex, higher-order functions of the top of the brain, the PFC. It's from this seat that you can redirect bad habits, make better choices, create new routines, spur your creative juices, and enjoy all of the sensual pleasures life has to offer, including sex. This capacity to direct your life is what makes up your operational intelligence.

Operational intelligence involves learning how to own our feelings of anger, for example, listen to what fuels these feelings, acknowledge our interpretations and expectations, and then take appropriate action (if necessary) to remedy the issue. In other words, negative feelings are fine feelings to have. You don't want to deny or block them. But you also want to shift to view these feelings as opportunities to become even more connected and intimate instead of reeling or free falling in defense mode.

Operational intelligence is, in essence, the process that enables us to realize that we all have the inner resources that we need to be happy. Here's an example. The old version of you is based on you not liking your body. You think, "If I lose weight, then I will be happy. Then I will want to have sex again and feel good in and out of clothes." So you diet, fight your feelings of hunger and cravings for comfort foods. You deprive yourself. Lose a few pounds. You feel good for a bit, but then get stressed about something and eat more. You then feel discouraged, fat, and unhappy. And, even if you manage to lose the weight, something else bugs you. You don't like the stretch marks, or your wrinkles, or your job, or something else. And then it's onto the next goal that you think will make you happy.

The new version of you would start with: "I like my body. I want to worship my body. I want to feed myself delicious healthy foods. I want to move my body in ways that feel good. I consciously step into loving my body exactly as it is. I decide to be happy in my body." From here, you listen to your body and feed it foods that taste good and are good for you. You dance, you play, you move your body because it feels good. You enjoy your body. You feel sexy. You want to share your beautiful body with your lover. You focus on self-love and self-soothing and self-care.

Let's take a look at how to put this self-care into action.

Creating a New Recipe

Janet is a good example of how to become an intelligent user of your own operational intelligence. I use an approach with Janet that harnesses the power of her imagination and inner resources to create the solutions for the challenges that she is facing. Putting together and improvising a number of different strategies I learned in trainings such as NLP, Ericksonian hypnotherapy, and personal growth workshops, as well as my own experiences in psychotherapy, I have created an exercise I call "cooking up a new recipe."

The first step in this process involves helping Janet get into a relaxed, receptive state in which she can access her creative self and find new directions for the future. I suggest that she bring her attention and awareness inward, focus on her breathing, and then give herself full permission "to be exactly as she is and for the moment to be exactly as it is." This inward-facing reflection will help bring to the surface thoughts and feelings that typically stay below our conscious awareness.

This permission acts as a powerful suggestion that helps to soften our tensions, whether they be psychological or physical — something I learned during a training at Harvard's Mind Body Institute years ago. Once Janet is relaxed and receptive, I explain how she can reconfigure her way of being and create new outcomes for herself.

Specifically, I say to her:

> At some point in the past you were very much in touch with your
> own erotic and playful energies. There's still a sliver of your old

erotic self buried just beneath the surface. Let's imagine the you on the other side of this challenge. Visualize and sense the you who has gotten back her groove, the future you who is feeling turned on by life, turned on sexually, turned on by a man who loves you, enlivened creatively, inspired by living and loving fully and freely.

Janet surprises herself by being able to vividly imagine her future self:

> It was like a delicious daydream. I saw myself becoming a yoga teacher, opening up my own studio, becoming a holistic mindfulness practitioner, and becoming a very sexy, playful, enthusiastic lover of life.

Janet has come up with her own new recipe for her future self.

Janet then grounds this new recipe in her body by making a practice audio tape she can use to reinforce these messages, and even more importantly, to train herself to pay attention to how she can put this recipe into action. She begins to use Yogic breath exercises, including working with the pelvic floor (a technique called Mula Bhanda or Root Lock; see page 150).

Breath work calms the nervous system, which enables us to access our underlying systems and experience the feelings themselves. The more that we elicit the parasympathetic system, the more relaxed and receptive we will be to new suggestions for ourselves, signaling to our brain's defensive systems that we are safe. Breath exercises also allow us to harness our emotional attention and wake up the deep pelvic muscles, which are so important for good sex. Bringing any kind of blood flow to the genitals will increase our potential for orgasm. I generally teach this tool to people with sex issues, but it is good for all kinds of scenarios in which we need to downregulate our defensive systems and open ourselves up to new ways of being.

....

Good Sex Tool: Breath Basics

1. Breathe in and out through nostrils — long small inhale; longer smooth exhalation (making out breath longer than inhalation strengthens parasympathetic tone by engaging vagal brake/enhances cardiac variability — which promotes heart health).

2. Pay attention to gentle pauses — when lungs are filled — both at top of breath before wave of exhalation and at bottom before next wave of inhalation (tuning into sensation of gravity) is initiated. Bringing the mind to them has a calming effect.

....

Janet begins to create a repository of "wins" in each new behavior that she adopts. Wins are simply positive things she thinks, does, or creates based on her new recipe. Who decides when something is a win? Rather than looking for validation extrinsically, she focuses on being the source of her own approval. She likes the vibe of the folks at the yoga studio and takes a risk to invite some of the other students out for coffee. This is a big win for Janet: to ask for what she wants without apology. Soon Janet starts getting interested in dating, and sex, again — at least sex with herself. "I've started masturbating again," she tells me one winter afternoon as we sip tea in my office. Another big win. "I think that is a good sign," she observes. And I totally agree. Janet's appetite for sexual pleasure has reignited — because she now feels safe and has become un-frozen. Her natural sexual desire reasserts itself as an extension of her self-care.

She understands that creating new emotional habits takes time, and that after thirty, sixty, or ninety days, she will have laid down the seeds of new habits. To reinforce this new habit she keeps track of her wins in her journal, celebrating both little and big wins. But at this point, the recipe is formulated to rebalance what is out of whack in the basement.

It will be a journey for Janet, one that will take time and patience. But she is moving toward feeling that she doesn't have to wait to lose weight to reenter the world of relating. And it all starts with her relationship with herself. Janet becomes consciously able to self-nurture. As she explains, "I check in three times a day with me. I write in my journal about what's on my mind, what I am feeling in my body, and what my emotional weather is like in that moment. And I always end with asking myself, 'What do I want?'"

Janet's journey began when she became attuned to her PANIC-CARE imbalance. She began to feel a tremendous sense of relief: she finally made sense to herself. She also grew to appreciate that her imbalance was not her fault, and that she could take steps to consciously repair her attachment style. Then Janet's new ways to be — "her recipe" — also meant that she was able to revise her self-image to include being *entitled, worthy, deserving, lovable, and self-loving*. This helped her harness the power of her cognitive (top brain) attention and consciously guide herself into choosing to be these ways, such as taking more time and energy for self-care, studying yoga, and learning how to ask for what she wanted. One important aspect of her self-care regimen was learning to say no and asserting healthy boundaries with people, so that she could not be taken advantage of.

As a result, she was able to cultivate a more secure relationship with herself and the world. Once Janet's PANIC/GRIEF system came into balance, her PLAY and LUST systems could reboot. Janet's journey from being at the mercy of her bottom brain's emotional imbalances to finally arriving at a place where she can apply her own operational intelligence to create change embodies the ultimate transformation and her refinding of pleasure in all ways.

Using OI to Transform Your Relationship

So far we have considered the impact that imbalances of core emotional systems have on one individual. Now let's take a look at what happens when two people with significant imbalances in the emotional basement attempt to have a long-term relationship. Consider the case of Beth and Richard. It's Wednesday afternoon on an uncharacteristically warm and sunny winter afternoon. Beth and Richard are seated in my home office, looking tense and shutdown. A couple with a track record of eight years of chaos, they're here to tackle a stormy relationship characterized by big highs and bigger lows. I think of Richard Burton and Liz Taylor when I think of them — all the fighting, fucking, fleeing, and reuniting. Ironically, both had left secure marriages in which they had grown bored. They got hooked on the chemistry of drama until it became unsustainable.

From a neuroscience perspective, the excitement of "unpredictability and uncertainty" (prediction reward error plus novelty) was driving the dopamine "SEEKING" pump and prolonging their new relationship energy (and the corresponding neurochemicals) until the process imploded upon itself, with one too many fights, which led to the current state of midrelationship agony.

With some coaching from me (following their biggest blowup to date), they had been doing better: cultivating the skills of an effective relationship. Emboldened by their progress, they started planning to move in together and blending their respective families in small doses — taking small but significant steps like meeting relatives who had yet to be met — and ultimately honing a much healthier, more conscious way of relating. But as the drama seemed to soften, they managed to skip scheduling regular therapy sessions that no longer seemed so pressing, as holidays and sick kids and other considerations took precedence.

Then a new bout of distress arose, on the heels of a major business setback for Richard. When triggered by fear (in the case of Richard — fear of losing his job, fear of losing control of his career, fear of being out of control in general), he, like most people, goes on emotional autopilot, which for him looks like shutting down, tuning out, and turning off. At his core, similar to Janet, Richard has an imbalance in the PANIC/GRIEF system (due to an alcoholic mother who was abusive to him during childhood), which shows up as Richard retreating when he gets increasingly anxious. Richard's withdrawal greatly triggers Beth, whose own emotional template of fear and anxiety looks like her PANIC system is in overdrive: she becomes hypervigilant, makes furtive phone calls, constantly checks in with Richard, and when he is around, becomes smothering. Both are ramping up their defenses, albeit in almost opposite ways, in a reverberating system heading south.

So what tools do they use individually and as a couple to reboot their pleasure system? First, we need to address the "bio" part of the bio/psycho/social approach. They need to calm down their brain-bodies before we can get anything accomplished. For this, some basic breath work is in order. My favorite go-to calming breath is called "ujjayi," or ocean breath. It is very simple. I have them breathe in and out through the nostrils, making the sound of the ocean, and extending the out breath just a bit longer than the inhalation. The key here is to slow down the breath in general and extend the exhalation just a bit longer than the inhalation, which triggers the stress responses mediated by the autonomic nervous system (ANS) to slow down and the "alarm" system to turn off. Regular practice of this simple breath tool actually strengthens the calming, restorative portion of the ANS — the parasympathetic division, which, by the way, is a necessary physiological state that make male erections possible.

Once they are calm, we begin learning an important interpersonal communication tool with the knowledge that we can always return to the ujjayi breath if anxiety arises.

I have them take turns listening to each other through parts 1 and 2 of the Active Listening processes (see opposite for part 2, and page 121 for part 1), which has the potential to supercharge your attention to sensations. (You might become aware of a tightness in the chest, tension in the hands or legs, a lump in the throat.) Richard and Beth listen to their own bodies and put their sensations into words in order to ground and connect. The goal is to tolerate the physical sensations sufficiently for them to peak and release — along with the emotions driven by the triggered defensive systems. Then and only then, by coming to their senses, do they recognize how hijacked they are by the overactivation of their defensive systems (FEAR for Richard and PANIC for Beth).

They begin to see how their anxious attachment styles present in different ways: Richard withdraws into his anger while Beth becomes clingy and smothering. Next, they observe how their pattern of relationship drama (fight, fuck, flee) reinforces the defenses and eventually shuts down the PLAY and LUST energies. Then, they are ready to use some top-down operational intelligence to reframe their response.

As the sessions progress, they are able to access the CARE systems and participate in a very constructive discussion. This not only allows them to witness their habitual behaviors, but also gives me the opportunity to translate what they report into what is happening in their emotional operating systems — and how they can better operate them.

Both Richard and Beth had to figure out what they want as opposed to what they do not want. I ask them, "Why are you here? What outcome do you want?"

They agree that they both want to feel love, care, and yes, lust toward each other again. They want to stop the fighting and the drama. With that as their North star, they then figure out strategies for their particular "recipe" and redesign the ways they interact. They will both, as individuals, need a new way of envisioning their relationship and future together, and this begins with rebalancing their respective emotional systems and then using a conscious idea of how to move forward as a couple. (See page 97 for Reframing Your Outcomes exercise.)

After Richard and Beth clearly see what they want to create, they can use their conscious commitments to guide their behavior and choices, which in the past have been subject to nonconscious patterns and out-of-whack emotional systems. Similar to Janet, Richard and Beth first need to focus on soothing the PANIC/GRIEF system before they can establish a more healthy, hedonic dynamic. They must foster a deep understanding of how the imbalances affect them, train themselves to feel the emotions but not get hijacked by them, and then consciously guide their attention to creating "wins" in the areas they want to change.

....

Good Sex Tool: Active Listening, part 2

This exercise further enhances your ability to validate your partner's emotional experience. We all have an urgent need to be heard and to be felt. The ability of our partners not to just hear our words but to reflect on and hear our feelings is critical for good relating. The roots of emotional intelligence rely on both our ability to identify our own emotions and also accurately interpret other people's emotional states. We then need to effectively learn to communicate about our feelings in order to be able to meet the needs that are driving these emotions. Sometime in the context of relationships, we may be the cause—or at least the trigger of—our partner's less than warm-and-fuzzy feelings. It may be difficult for us to hear, acknowledge, and tolerate these emotions because they trigger our own feelings, especially if we feel responsible. This exercise allows for space to speak and to listen, and it is very helpful in fostering a more trusting connection between partners.

For example, during a session, a husband might be telling his wife about some difficulties that he's having with her being less available due to a demanding work schedule. The wife might say, "Based on what you have been expressing, I imagine that you might be feeling frustrated, lonely, sad, or even angry with me? Is that correct?"

The ability to hear into the emotions underlying our partner's words is extremely powerful. The speaker gets to then correct by elaboration if the partner is on target or not. Often you can tell very quickly by watching the speaker's nonverbal reaction whether he or she feels "gotten." And it feels incredibly good to be gotten.

Steps

1. Listener to speaker: "Given that you say _____, I imagine that you might be feeling __. Is that correct?"

2. Speaker: "Yes — and furthermore ____" (speaker can elaborate if desired). Or "No, that isn't correct. How I am actually feeling is ____."

3. At which point, the Listener tries again to put into words how he/she thinks the Speaker is feeling until it's clear.

....

Physical Good Sex Tools to Rebalance Your Body, Your Emotions, and Your Relationships

As you've seen through the stories we've explored so far, the ability to rediscover your capacity for pleasure is not just possible but probable. Each of you individually and as couples have the capacity to create your own recipe, using your operational intelligence in your life, sexual and otherwise.

As you've read through the stories of various clients and how they resolved their emotional disruptions in order to address their anhedonia and bring their sexual and sensual pleasures back online, you've encountered numerous tools — those that address your personal emotional imbalances and those that help you reconnect with yourself or your partner. From visualization exercises, unpacking your anger, and determining your attachment style to active listening and scheduling playdates, these tools can help you in an immediate, accessible way. What follows are additional tools that will help you resuscitate your pleasure pathway. These begin with exercises that help you relax your body. As we've seen, you will be much more open to pleasure and connection when you feel safe, comfortable, and relaxed. The second group of tools work at a more cognitive level, enabling you to reframe how your emotions may or may not be helping you.

GOOD SEX TOOL: MULA BHANDAS

By raising awareness and bringing blood flow to the pelvic region, you connect your breath to a pleasure center. This is what is known as a Mula Bhanda exercise. It begins with Breath Basics (page 142) and then adds in the next two steps:

1. Take a long smooth inhalation.
2. Just as you begin the exhalation, gently contract the anal sphincter and hold.
3. Next, lift the floor of the pelvis in the same kind of action you use to stop the flow of urine. I call this "pulling up on the floor of the pelvis," including the perineum (area between genitals and anus). Gently hold this as you breathe out a bit more.
4. Then, contract the lower abdominal muscles and pull the navel in toward the spine — and hold this also as the outbreath continues.
5. Lastly, drop your chin to chest and release the last of the exhalation.
6. Then release the breath and the energy locks.
7. Breathe regularly for a few breaths and then repeat steps.
8. Finally — take a few minutes to soak up the benefits of the practice.

This exercise can be extremely helpful in learning how to calm an overactive "monkey" mind. An incredible and unexpected side effect of this practice is that it can supercharge the sexual response and also rebalance sexual energy that is too high or too low. Indeed, there's tons of scientific evidence that doing these kinds of yoga and breath exercises can reap big benefits to our physical, emotional, and sexual well-being. Working with the floor of the pelvis in this way can also strengthen the muscles of the floor of the pelvis and abdomen, help increase our ability to orgasm, and overall balance what is out of balance neurochemically.

GOOD SEX TOOL: NOTICE AND IMAGINE SENSATIONS

Many of the Good Sex Tools are designed to connect your brain to your body, so that you can feel the pleasure in a visceral, tangible way. This exercise helps you to focus internally and become very clear about what you are feeling in your own body at any given time. This ability to tune into your sensations prepares you for more full-bodied pleasure, sexual and otherwise.

1. Sit down in a comfortable chair.
2. Close your eyes and begin to do a mental body scan from your head down to your toes, stopping to become aware of each area of your body.
3. When you notice an ache, in your hip for instance, imagine why your hip is aching. From sitting too long at your desk? From too long of a walk in uncomfortable shoes? If you feel, for instance, that you have a slight headache or some stomach upset — again try and imagine the cause for the feeling.

Use this exercise to become familiar with the habits and sensations of your body and learn to cue into the possible roots of these sensations.

GOOD SEX TOOL: YOGA

Yoga has a direct, positive effect on many aspects of the pleasure pathway. Many yoga poses, or asanas (as they are called), work the muscles in your core—all of which enhance sexual functioning. The toning and strengthening of the muscles in the hips, stomach, butt, and groin all support better sensation, sexual response, and orgasm. Yoga exercise gives particular emphasis to the perineum, otherwise known as the pelvic floor (the muscle between the anus and genitals). These are the muscles that deliver the sensation of pleasure, especially during sex. They contract spontaneously during orgasm! Stimulating, strengthening, and stretching these muscles increases blood flow, which improves responsiveness. Women benefit from doing these exercises for more reasons than just sexual pleasure! Indeed, strengthening the entire pelvic floor supports overall uterine health, wards off incontinence, and supports organs. A regular yoga practice also increases body "awareness," which means simply that it allows the mind to become more aware of the body and thus feel more of its physical sensations, and more acutely. Several studies show how both men and women can "improve all domains of sexual function" through yoga. In addition, yoga for men has been shown to increase levels of testosterone, the hormone that drives male libido. It's well known that yoga is restorative and following a regular yoga practice will energize and relax your body, improve your immune system, lower your heart rate, and increase your overall well-being. People with a renewed sense of energy are more likely to engage in sexual activity.

Working with these physical tools is what helps us be receptive, ready, and responsive to the next phase: reframing your outcomes.

The Power of Suggestion: Gestalt Approach to Rebalance your Systems

Are you aware of how much of our time throughout the day is spent in trance? We naturally fall into a kind of altered state every time our mind wanders, or we are doing something without our full conscious awareness. Our brain has an enormous capacity to repeat well-known pathways of behavior, which enables us to do things like drive all the way to the office or gym without even thinking about where we are going. Similarly, our symptoms of distress are unwanted spontaneous trance symptoms. We mostly suggest negative stuff to ourselves below the radar as "automatic thoughts."

Early on in my career, I was fortunate enough to work with "big, bad" Brad Blanton, PhD, the author of the *Radical Honesty* series. He humorously describes himself as white trash with a PhD. Blanton suggests that most of human suffering comes from our simply not being in our truth from moment to moment. He says that although we think that we lie to protect others, we are actually trying to protect ourselves, and in the long run sabotaging our ability to be present and joyful. What truly underlies our fear of telling the truth, Blanton suggests, is that it might feel too good and feeling *too* good is terrifying to most of us.

Much of my approach to leading clients out of anhedonia and back on the path to pleasure has emerged from a combination of my early training in Gestalt psychotherapy and the work I learned from Brad. Gestalt teaches us to complete our incomplete emotional experiences. We tend to truncate our emotional expressions because of societal messages that train parents, peers, and eventually ourselves to shut down. It is essential for us to learn to tolerate our emotions such that they can be fully experienced, peak, and then be released. Those overly defensive emotions that stay locked in our memories are actually more problematic than the fully expressed ones. We need to get mad enough to get over it, sad enough to get over it, scared enough to get over it, and even joyful enough to get over it. Key to this is becoming aware of our body's sensations and moving away from reliance on cognitive thoughts.

We can harness the power of our own attention by bringing awareness inward with and through the suggestions of Ericksonian language both with and without inducing trance. You can do these exercises (below) on your own at home or in an otherwise safe, comfortable environment. These exercises are also designed to help you distinguish between what happened versus our interpretation of what happened. How we see things often tinges the actual experience or its meaning, and this is how we become more responsible for creating our own emotional experiences. This may seem kind of simplistic, and it is. The whole point is to move out of our heads and get more in touch with our experiences such that we don't get controlled by our overactive minds making up all kinds of interpretations! Our stories become more important than our experiences, which then get in the way of actually connecting with ourselves and others.

I often use this approach with clients so they can become aware of their tendency to infuse what actually happens with their interpretations, which are usually influenced by imbalanced emotional systems. For example, people in a defensive mindset interpret messages from partners as threatening. They are in the FEAR or PANIC mind. As it is said, we always know what's on our minds, but we don't always know which mind we are in. The three exercises below — Notice and Imagine, Gestalt Hot Seat, and Gestalt Life Story — are similar in their structure. They ask you to tell and repeat your details or a significant event from your life in dramatic detail and then progressively more objectively, losing the drama, the emotional edge, and ultimately the interpretation.

As you tell and retell your story, shortening it and lessening the emotional flavors, you are discharging distress about what happened to you. The story becomes a less emotional version of what happened and more influenced by where you are now. There is empirical evidence that every time we retrieve a memory from long-term storage, it becomes fragile in the sense that we can intentionally alter it by updating the remembered experience from the vantage point of being more empowered and at choice about how we view what happened in the past. Ultimately, you can use this as a tool to help you stay present and release the past.

GOOD SEX TOOL: NOTICE AND IMAGINE

There's a huge difference between what we observe and what we imagine, which is an interpretation. We human beings are meaning-making, storytelling machines, which works pretty well most of the time, but we like to add our own "becauses" which are not always accurate in the end.

This is a fun way to try and establish the difference between what you're actually seeing and your interpretations of what you're observing. First, you state what you see or observe and then state what you imagine to be the reason behind the observation.

Sit across from your partner and you say:

"I notice _____ and I imagine _____."

This could be "I notice you are wearing pants," and "I imagine that you're wearing pants because you're cold."

"I noticed that you have glasses on," and "I imagine that you wear glasses because you have some kind of astigmatism."

"I notice that you have hair, and I imagine it's because you're a mammal."

As we become better attuned at noticing and then recognizing that we jump to all sorts of conclusions (interpretations), often at the expense of being present to what is actually going on, we can develop new habits that help us check in with our partners, rather than staying stuck in our "imaginings." For example, you are out to dinner with your partner, and you're sharing details about a challenging development at work. You notice your partner seems "distracted." Ordinarily you might interpret this as disinterest or even judgment. But rather than jumping into an old habit of interpretation and building up a head of steam about how "he

should be more attentive," you might simply lean over and say, "I notice that you are looking away and I imagine that you might be annoyed,
bored, or disinterested." Your partner then gets a chance to clarify what
he is experiencing. He might be hungry, tired, or even horny. He might
not even be aware of his what's on his mind — or what mind he's in —
until you create this opportunity to go deeper.

Clarifying our interpretations of observations is an important step
toward recognizing that very often we are making up all sorts of stories
about what we're seeing right in front of us.

GOOD SEX TOOL: GESTALT HOT SEAT

This exercise is typically done in front of a group of people because there
is an emphasis on speaking aloud and having witnesses. There is tons of
evidence that sharing our concerns with others has a multitude of health
benefits — and conversely just thinking about our concerns without
expressing tends to only make things worse. And what could be better
than having a bunch of dedicated listeners paying good attention to you!
However, you can do this exercise with a close friend or your partner, or
even by yourself. The crux of the exercise is enabling you to reexperience
your old memories while you refeel the feelings you associate with the
event.

As you tell the story of the particular event that has affected you
(rather than your whole life story, which you will do below), you want to
notice what is going on for you: What feelings rise to the surface? How is
your body responding to these feelings? As you feel the feelings in your
body, allow the accompanying emotions to peak and release so they become unstuck.

For the Gestalt Hot Seat, bring to mind a particular event that you
consider traumatic or significant, and then recount the episode or event
in detail.

In each retelling, take away emotional modifiers and add in any background information that you now are aware of. Here's an example:

1. Lodged in your memory is an image of your sister being thrown against the wall by your enraged father, with you cowering behind the bed and your mother screaming at the top of her lungs. For years you bring this image and scenario to mind each time you think of how your childhood was filled with abuse, violence, and neglect.

2. Now, you begin to retell this story: You see your father (who was out of work) lose his temper at your sister, who happened to be at the wrong place at the wrong time. Your mother feels helpless so all she can do is scream. You are little — five or six — and crouch in the corner so as to stay out of the way.

3. When you next retell the story, you see your farther as supremely frustrated with work, his marriage, and himself. You see your mother as having no sense of her inner resources to change her situation. Both your parents are stuck in old behaviors that do not reflect who they are as people. You and your sister are innocent bystanders impacted by two adults who have not evolved.

4. Eventually the story becomes that your parents were up to their eyeballs in stressors for which they were poorly prepared, and they lacked sufficient support to help them cope.

5. Add another level of perspective: the story winds down to the conclusion that you learned many lessons from their mistakes, which have made you the wonderful insightful self-regulating person you have become.

6. And the bottom line is that you now have all of the resources internally to create all of the resources you need
   to live and love.

GOOD SEX TOOL: GESTALT LIFE STORY

In this exercise, you will use the same retelling technique but create an arc that encompasses your entire life. Again, although this technique is typically practiced in front of a group, you can adapt it by writing it out in your journal, taping it on your smartphone or other recording device, or asking your partner or other significant person in your life to listen.

The point here is to take the high points — or low points — of your own story and repeat its sequence of events until you remove its emotional charge.

In each rendering of your story, you make the telling more objective, less dramatic, and less emotionally laden. You peel away the layers until you see it starkly. Eventually, as you practice, you can shorten the story until it is a brief one with you as the amazing hero — you lived to tell!

GOOD SEX TOOL: JOURNALING

This tool may seem all too familiar — but it is still a powerful way to get at what thoughts and feelings lurk underneath. Indeed, research unequivocally supports the notion that writing has a powerful positive impact on our emotional well-being and the overall health of the immune system. In my practice, I've seen how the act and process of putting the thoughts in your head into words on the page is an immensely powerful tool for understanding how you think and feel. Free writing in particular allows you to witness what is on the top of the mind and what lurks beneath. It is simply about dumping what is on the mind onto the page without any editing or structure.

As you begin to write regularly, you can also become aware of the cognitive distortions that creep into your mind from the midlevel memories. It's especially helpful to distinguish between what we feel in our bodies and what we think we are feeling emotionally. Suddenly, "I'm fine" becomes "I guess I'm anxious because I feel a tightness in my chest." There are always physical sensations that go along with emotions, but it takes training to know what we actually think or believe and what is an old or outdated interpretation of what's going on.

This tool can be used as part of a regular self-care practice to always have a sense of what's on your mind, what's going on in your body, and what's going on in your emotional basement. By fostering healthy self-attunement, you are more likely to keep your seven core emotions in good balance.

Hopefully, you have found many of these Good Sex Tools not only helpful but also enjoyable; they are designed to connect your body and brain in ways that open you to your innate drive for pleasure. They are also designed to be entry points to your core emotions and your layers of unconscious habits, putting you back into balance if necessary. Together, these tools will help you bring balance to your core emotions and:

- Recruit SEEKING
- Dampen FEAR
- Tamp down RAGE
- Soothe PANIC/GRIEF
- Balance CARE
- Boost PLAY
- Resuscitate LUST

In the next chapter, you will take another step toward your pleasure-filled future by learning how to address your sexual desires and lingering limitations straight on. When we get the full scoop on all of the moving pieces that impact our sexuality — from how our bodies and brains are shaped by genetics and biology, to how sexual desire is more than simply being horny or not, and how our unique erotic fingerprints or sexual styles can mesh with our partners or at times clash — we will see that our sexuality is a vast, delicious, and highly misunderstood arena for continued learning, growth, and of course, the promise of good sex!

8

Sex as a Tool for Transformation

One of the most powerful dimensions of sex is that it's not only a window into who we are but can be an actual tool for transformation. In the last several chapters, you dived deep into your emotional core, coming away with a keener sense of where your imbalances may lie and the appropriate recipe for reframing what you want in your life. This bio/psycho/social approach is a key component for accessing your pleasure pathway. However, some women and men, as couples or individuals, find it easier to deal directly with the sexual issues and then discover that their emotional imbalances even out on their own. So wherever you may be in your journey with yourself or your partner, know that there is no right way to approach your emotional or sexual issues — inevitably you will likely encounter both.

In this chapter, you will use what you now know about yourself to return to your sexual desire set point and further discover your "erotic fingerprint." This and other tools will help you take a closer look at your satisfaction with sex, how you match up with that of your partner, if you are in a relationship, and how you can take further steps to embrace all that good sex has to offer you.

The Sex and Gender Continuum

We tend to view sex as binary, either male or female, but for nature, sex is expressed more richly, on a nuanced, complex continuum. And gender, how feminine or masculine a person is, has very complicated bio/psycho/social roots. For starters, consider the distinction between sex and gender: Sex is biological — what we mean by "male" or "female." Gender is more of a bio/psycho/social construct, which includes not only things that might be biologically influenced, but also what an individual's learning (psycho) and society (social) establish as appropriately "masculine" or "feminine." Let's focus on the bio portion of the equation. There are three levels of our biological sex: chromosomal, gonadal, and hormonal. At the moment of conception, the male sperm determines our *chromosomal* sex (by either contributing an X or a Y gene to fertilize the egg, which contains only an X chromosome), resulting in a female (XX) or male (XY). Early in development, the gonads (future ovaries or testes) remain undifferentiated, with both sexes having two sets of precursor "ducts" or basic plumbing that can develop into the necessary organs (Wolfian equals "male" and Mullerian equals "female"). At this early point, all fetal genitalia appear female.

Going forward, for males, if development continues normally, at about six weeks after conception, the gonads (testes) begin to develop (*gonadal sex*) in response to genetic signals. The testes then start to secrete testosterone (*hormonal sex*), which is transformed by an enzyme into dihydrostestosterone (DHT), which functions to masculinize the sex organs, causing the deterioration of the "female" Mullerian duct system and the proliferation of the masculine precursors (Wolfian ducts), culminating in the masculinization of the external genitals, a process which occurs between nine and twelve weeks in utero.

In chromosomal females it is the *absence* of a cue (since there is no Y chromosome) that signals the development of the Mullerian ducts into what will become the female sex organs and genitalia and cause the deterioration of the masculine Wolfian duct precursors.

The brain, on the other hand, is a whole different story. In males it is masculinized in a completely different step during which testosterone is converted into estrogen. This results in the development of a preponderance of places in the brain sensitive to testosterone, and the reason why males tend to "have sex on the brain" more often than females. Who knew that it takes a female hormone to make a male brain!

The question becomes: if estrogen is responsible for the masculinization of the male brain, how does it not have a similar effect on the developing female brain? As it turns out, the developing female brain is insulated from the "masculinizing" effects of estrogen by special proteins that are manufactured under the direction of the XX chromosomes. Hence, if there isn't a Y chromosome driving the process, the brain's default is to be feminized. But this isn't as passive a process as it may sound. It is through an active suppression of certain key enzymes that otherwise would kick in and cause the brain to be masculinized that the female brain prevails. And the female brain significantly differs from the male in having way more circuits sensitive to the "tend and befriend" hormone oxytocin.

Since the brain and body are "sexed," as it were, in two separate, independent steps, things might not always unfold as nature intended. During the course of development, biological factors can derail the regularly scheduled "program" and result not in just two "sexes" (i.e., male brain-body and female brain-body) but also other combinations. It is

possible to have a male brain/female body or female brain/male body —
hence four "sexes" in total. Some cultures actually have accommodated
and acknowledge these variations in sex and gender.

To complicate matters further, the maleness and femaleness of the
brain exists on a continuum — meaning that it is not an all-or-nothing
process. Some brains may be more masculinized or feminized than others, since both sexes have both kind of circuits — just in different ratios.
And we haven't even addressed the instances when the genetic, chromosomal sex is other than XX or XY. This information may explain some
instances in which a person feels "trapped" in a body that doesn't match
the sex of their "mind," such as is the case with people who identify as
transgender. The variability of how the brain is "sexed" during development may also play a role in the variability of sexual orientation as well.
In sum, nature loves diversity, but culture isn't quite so fond of it.

Men and Women Are Indeed Different:
"Sex on the Brain" Versus "Tend and Befriend"

An important starting point for understanding sexual desire is to appreciate that hormones play a key role in motivating our sexual appetites
and behaviors. In fact the operation of our sexual systems depends on a
cascade of hormones that affect us at two critical points during our life
cycle — initially during the course of embryonic development (these are
called "organizing" effects, which establish the architecture of the brain/
body) and later on, when we hit puberty (these are the "activating" effects, which turn on the wired-in systems).

Most people don't know that the "masculinization" of the brain and
body happen during embryonic development at two distinct and separate points, facilitated by two different hormones, which has huge potential in clarifying some issues involving sexual orientation, gender

identification, and transgenderism (in which the "sex" of the brain does not apparently match that of the body). As far as the "activating" effects of the hormones, we know that the hormone testosterone is responsible for the sex drive in both male and female mammals and people. What is not usually discussed (but has been well established) is that testosterone has more impact on the male mammalian brain.

While it might be considered politically incorrect to call attention to fundamental differences in how male and female brains are wired, modern neuroscience has provided tons of evidence to support that there are indeed significant differences. Although it is true that the brain of each sex has some "feminine" and some "masculine" networks or circuits, if all goes according to plan in the process of embryological development, male brains simply have more places for the testosterone (and another hormone related to testosterone, vasopressin) to work — by connecting with structures called receptors activated by the hormones. The "receptive fields" or places for testosterone to have influence are plentiful in the male brain. This feature explains the general finding that males tend to report having "sex on the mind" more frequently than females.

On the other hand, if all goes well during embryonic development, the female brain comes equipped with sufficient receptors sensitive to the hormone oxytocin — the hormone that is associated with decreased anxiety, increased trust, and social bonding. Oxytocin affects male brains similarly but there are substantially fewer oxytocin circuits in the male brain. Interestingly enough, the female sex hormone estrogen turns up the activity of the oxytocin circuits in the brain, while testosterone in the male brain fires up the vasopressin circuits, fueling competition and sexual interest.

Another fascinating aspect of female sexuality is that women's interest in the erotic can wax and wane in response to cyclical changes in brain chemistry. At peak fertility, when estrogen and progesterone levels are high, some women report more sexual thoughts and fantasies. Studies have also shown that women engage in more sexual behavior during their fertile periods (with rates of intercourse rising by 24 percent during the six days flanking ovulation). But way more than biology affects female sexuality. One need only read the fascinating research done by Dr. Meredith Chivers, a colleague from Queens University in Ontario, who has demonstrated that, in women, arousal of the genitals (as measured by blood flow in response to audiovisual erotic stimuli) simply doesn't translate into subjective sexual arousal or feeling turned on. In other words, blood flow to female genitals tends to be a nonspecific response to all sorts of erotic stimuli, regardless of the female participant's sexual orientation, which doesn't necessarily correlate with "feeling turned on." Blood flow to the women's genitals increases when the participants watched males with females, males with males, females with females, and even bonobos (those randy pygmy chimpanzees) getting it on.

This type of arousal is keenly different from how male arousal works: men's genitals only rise to the occasion, so to speak, in response to stimuli matching their own sexual orientation. And for men, increased blood flow to the penis in this type of study usually translates into increased subjective turn on. This explains why Viagra-type drugs don't work for women. With these drugs, you can indeed increase blood flow to the female genitals, but it doesn't do much for the ladies in terms of either subjective (experienced) arousal or desire. Suffice it to say that sexuality for women appears to have more complex underpinnings, which are not as well understood.

Men and women also experience some aspects of sex differently. At first, in the early days, sexuality research by Masters and Johnson (1966), Kaplan (1979), and Lief (1977) described the sexual response cycle as a linear process that begins with desire/arousal, moves to a plateau or middle stage of intensified arousal or excitement, and then on to a third stage of orgasm and/or ejaculation. We have moved beyond this model not only because women don't fit neatly into it but also because we know so much more about the varying ways that humans in general become aroused and experience desire.

Several sexologists, including Beverly Whipple and K. B. Brash-McGeer and Rosemary Basson, distinguish the female sexual response cycle as being more circular than linear because there are so many more dimensions to what drives female desire and arousal. Basson shifted the nonlinear model farther by emphasizing that women are not necessarily motivated by sex for the release of orgasm but rather "personal satisfaction," which may come through the emotional experience of intimacy with a partner. Essentially, for women, as compared with men, sexual desire might not be as driven by physically experienced "horniness" — but rather more motivated and accessed by and through the warm, intimate, and fuzzy partnership pathway.

Why are these models helpful or significant? Because they underscore that the pleasure of sex comes at different stages and in different forms: in the turn-on level of stimuli; in the predicted expectation that sex is going to happen; in the body-focused build-up of increased blood flow and muscle tension of the excitement and plateau stages; and ultimately in the release of the orgasm. If pleasure is experienced all along the way and is naturally variable, and the brain's involvement is paramount, then how we think about solving our sexual problems needs to consider these realities.

Spontaneous Versus Responsive Desire

The challenge of two people (regardless of their gender or sex) being in sync sexually is further complicated by another important sex difference: from the biological perspective, it appears that men are hardwired to have more robust "spontaneous" desire. This means they are simply "hornier" — tending to think about sex, fantasize about sex, and want to have sex more frequently on average than women. In contrast, women tend to have less "spontaneous desire" and higher levels of what is called "responsive" sexual desire, the type that lies beneath the surface and kicks in when the woman finds a partner appealing or becomes aroused through physical or emotional stimulation.

For men, desire more often just pops up, even before arousal — or simultaneously along with arousal. What often happens is that, over time in long-term relationships, women may experience a lower level of spontaneous desire than previously, and the partners may become concerned that the woman is suffering from low desire, when in fact, the responsive desire is there, below the surface, awaiting a kick-start. Just for the record, in some instances, it is the man who experiences the drop off of spontaneous desire, which can be even more disconcerting as that violates the expectation that men are "supposed" to have tons of sexual desire. When couples experience such disconnects, sometimes simply educating them about how desire works is all they need to get the sexual relationship back on track.

Men and women also tend to differ in their desire for more novelty; men want more novelty in sex in general, and also report wanting more sexual partners than women.

Bear in mind that all of these sex-related trends do not trump the many individual differences among men and women. There is great variation within each sex as to how these differences show up, not least of all because it is entirely possible that nature has wired some female brains to be organized more like male brains, and vice versa. And then we get to factor into the equation that our individual experiences with sexuality can vary tremendously (psycho), as can how we are socialized via our families, relationships, and cultures (social). All of these factors combine to affect our sexual attitudes, behaviors, and even preferences, such that the differences between the sexes become less salient than the sum total of an individual's bio/psych/social fingerprint. Yes — sex is indeed complicated!

The differences we have explored should help explain why men and women often tend to approach sex with different motivations and desires. One is not better than the other. Rather, for both women and men, understanding these essential differences helps to explain how or why couples can fall out of sync. It's also important to note that this plays out in all kinds of relationships, not just the traditional heterosexual partnerships. These individual bio/psycho/social fingerprints impact the sexual relationships of all individuals, whether they be gay, straight, bisexual, or gender queer (i.e., people who do not subscribe to traditional gender distinctions and may identify with both or neither gender). The bottom line is that our biological, psychological, and social factors interact and manifest in tremendous individual variability related to sexual desire and responsiveness.

The Rise and Inevitable Fall of New Relationship Energy

You know the honeymoon period of a relationship? That ecstatic, crazy-in-love period when all you want to do is rip each other's clothes off and screw your brains out? When you seem to be aroused by the mere sound of his voice? The scent of her perfume or skin? Sex during this phase is intense, passionate, and seems so, so easy (for most)! Then, after a few months or years, the excitement seems to wear off. You're no longer new to each other. Alas, some people even think they are no longer in love.

As mentioned earlier, what I've just described is the phenomenon called "new relationship energy," or NRE. And it eventually decreases and may even totally wear off. But it's not because people fall out of love; it's because the neurochemical cocktail that fuels the ecstatic feelings and nonstop lust naturally winds down. Over the past few years, researchers have begun to identify not only the brain areas related to NRE but also the neurochemicals involved.

What's going on when we are revved up on NRE? Dopamine is flooding our system and all we do is want, want, want. Sound familiar? At the same time, we are experiencing high levels of oxytocin and vasopressin, which help focus our attention on our connections and, in this instance, rev up our spontaneous desire — which is reinforced with ever more sensual contact. Even cortisol levels become elevated since falling in love is a kind of stressor as the individual goes through the concerns and potential insecurities about the new relationship. NRE is also associated with decreased levels of serotonin, queuing up the not-so-delightful tendency of ruminating that can be the dark side of NRE, where the person obsessively thinks about the partner (incidentally, people who suffer from obsessive-compulsive disorder tend to have lower levels of serotonin, which reverse after successful treatment).

Another finding is that levels of nerve growth factor, a neurotrophin (a protein involved in the survival, development, and function of brain cells), ramp up during the early passionate stages of love. It appears this is a kind of reaction to stress, too, and correlates with the highest ratings on the scales that rate our levels of passionate love.

NRE quickly ramps up our spontaneous desire to record highs (though our responsive desire remains intact) and then powerfully focuses our attention on the new lover — increasing our interest and motivation to get to know the person, find out if there is more than just chemistry in the attraction, and then ultimately settle in, if all goes well, to build a sustainable relationship. People with high levels of SEEKING, in particular, may be more susceptible to chasing the NRE buzz.

When people confuse NRE with love, they leave old comfortable partnerships for the excitement of the next hit of NRE. I always, always tell people not to make big decisions or operate heavy machinery while under the influence of the potent neuropeptides of NRE.

Eventually, with time, the process of habituation kicks in (think of it as a relationship variant of the hedonic treadmill), and the brain chemistry settles down. As we bond with the person, the CARE system takes over with its nutritious and satisfying (but not electrifying) neurochemicals. Our desire set point returns to baseline.

As NRE settles down, we may actually feel a big loss as we compare our ramped-up desire point relative to baseline. This is essentially what happens in the process of the desire curve. We forget about our original baseline desire and just compare the peak to what we experience after NRE resolves. We feel loss. We feel lack. Partners who enjoyed being pursued for sex feel abandoned when the sizzle subsides. Men whine that their female partners don't crave sex with them or want them anymore. Women feel deficient if they are no longer so intensely motivated to have sex. Even men can feel that their sexuality is somehow diminished as they return to baseline and are no longer fueled by the ramped-up LUST of NRE.

This inevitable variability—the movement from your emotional and sexual set point to a high point of NRE and then back down to your baseline, are what comprise your desire curve. This curve, represented by the graph on page 172, shows how your sexual baseline intersects with NRE, and also how men and women differ in regard to spontaneous/active desire and receptive/passive desire.

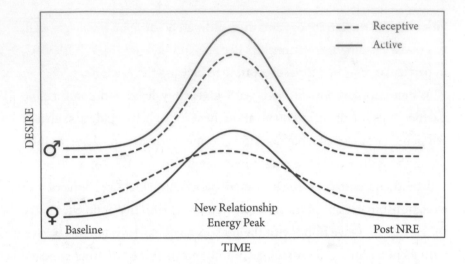

You will note that the general levels of spontaneous and receptive desire are higher, overall, for men. And for men, the receptive desire levels are quite similar to those of spontaneous desire. For both sexes, spontaneous desire peaks at the apex of NRE. For women, unlike men, the only time when spontaneous desire consistently exceeds receptive desire (other than during ovulation, which is not shown) is at peak NRE. For women, receptive desire is higher than spontaneous desire for most of the curve. And finally, for both sexes, you will notice that both spontaneous and receptive desire return to a baseline quite similar to that which preceded the NRE.

The critical point here is that you need to be aware of the flow of both spontaneous and receptive desire over the course of the desire curve — and recognize the tendency to forget about the original — baseline — desire set point. By recalling the original desire set point and comparing the post-NRE set point with the original, rather than comparing it with that at peak NRE, you will do much to counter the illusion that your return to baseline is an actual loss overall.

And there's another key dimension to understanding the dynamic nature of our LUST systems, especially when we are in relationships. We each have a unique erotic fingerprint, or sexual style, forged in part by our bio/psycho/social makeup, which can interact with our own and our partner's desire curve.

....

Good Sex Tool: Keep Track of Your Desire Set Point

As mentioned earlier, each of us, as a result of the combination of our biological, emotional, and relationship variables, has a desire "set point" that indicates how much spontaneous and receptive desire we tend to experience on *average*. This general range can vary in response to changes in circumstances and can shift over time. For example, for women, ovulation can temporarily dial up spontaneous desire. Starting a new relationship can powerfully ramp up spontaneous desire for both men and women for anywhere from eighteen to thirty-six months, or even longer if the partners don't have lots of access to each other. Factors such as increased anxiety or depression (imbalances in the core emotional systems) will cause a flattening of both spontaneous and responsive desire in the individual, as will experiencing loss and grief (PANIC/GRIEF systems activation). In addition, chronic, excessive stress will cause the defensive emotional systems to squash LUST plus PLAY. Recent studies show that simply not getting enough sleep will hamper sexual desire. And of course, physical illness will often put a kibosh on desire and lower the baseline set point.

Staying attuned to your body and its desire set point will help you anticipate natural fluctuations. Use these questions to tap into how you are feeling in terms of your sexual desire and LUST system.

1. How receptive are you to sex?

2. How often do you initiate sex?

3. How often do you masturbate?

4. How often do you fantasize about sex?

5. How much do you enjoy physical affection?

6. Do you think of yourself as desirous of sex?

7. Is it easy or hard for you to become aroused?

These questions are meant to simply help remind you of where you are at baseline, outside of NRE. (Refer back to page 171 for more details about your desire curve.)

What Is Your Erotic Fingerprint?

Regardless of whether we are in a relationship, we all have a certain sexual style. This style is not absolute or stagnant; it can change over time, just like we do. Sex therapist Sandra Pertot, PhD, first identified this concept by describing a number of "libido types" to help women and men understand their orientation around their own sexual desire and what makes them tick. I've modified some of Pertot's categories, added my own, and reconfigured them into what I call erotic fingerprints (EF), which I find helps my clients delve into the nature of their erotic selves. In addition, my fingerprint styles include biological dimensions that also incorporate temperament and natural desire set points, which are rooted in how active your LUST system is or where it is blocked by overactive defense systems (FEAR or RAGE), or hampered by imbalances in other core emotional systems such as CARE, PANIC/GRIEF, SEEKING, or PLAY).

Your erotic fingerprint also relates to your own psychological dimension and what midlevel-mind learnings may be left over from early trauma or other experiences that undermine your LUST or hinder your sexual expression. (Think shame that inhibits LUST — such as what Katie experienced.) Finally, my EF styles also include the bigger social climate (culture) and the specifics of where we are on the desire/relationship curve.

By identifying your erotic fingerprint, you gain insight into your sexual style and how you typically think about sex, experience sex, and desire sex. Knowing this information about yourself can help explain a possible disconnect with a spouse or current partner, or even when you have had trouble connecting with yourself.

I have identified seven basic erotic fingerprint styles for how people inhabit their own sexuality and relate to lovers. Take a look at the descriptions below. Where do you fit in? Are you a mix of a few styles? If you have a partner, can you recognize his or her fingerprint? As you read these descriptions, take note of how the different fingerprints mesh or collide with other styles.

THE SOULFUL LOVER

The Soulful Lover likes eye gazing, romance, and tender lovemaking. They are the touchy-feely type of lover, enjoying contact and closeness above all, and sometimes are not tuned into how his/her/their lover could be different. The Soulful Lover is also likely to be less sensitive to the desire curve shifts because they are more motivated by *connection* than sex itself. But, when it does come to sex, they will most likely be more keyed into responsive desire than suffer lots of ups and downs due to shifts in spontaneous desire. In general, the Soulful Lover may need more seduction before sex as it makes them feel more intimate with their partners. This could cause a problem if their partners don't initiate sex after the loss of NRE, making the Soulful Lover feel unwanted. If they tend to be anxious, they may pursue their partners for sex in order to feel close. If they tend toward low LUST and low PLAY for any reason, they may end up being more like the disinterested lover and just be available for sex in order to please the partner and seek closeness. Soulful Lovers are almost constitutionally allergic to partners who are explorers or more fixated on the intensity of sex and less into soft, tender lovemaking. For the Soulful Lover, wild and crazy sex may be less satisfying than sex that is focused on connection.

THE ROUGH-AND-TUMBLE LOVER

The Rough-and-Tumble hot sex lover feels it isn't really sex unless some furniture goes flying. This lover needs physically driven, athletic sex as a contact sport. In general, they don't mesh well with the kind of lover who needs soulful eye gazing and tender lovemaking. This kind of erotic fingerprint might be very affected by the drop in active desire that happens when NRE fizzles out. They tend to have high set points of active desire but may experience the post-NRE plunge as very upsetting. These people tend toward more dramatic internal experiences based on a kind of attachment to intensity. They get very tweaked in a negative way when their partner's unique erotic fingerprint might be less flexible post-NRE. This might happen, for example, when the tender Soulful Lover finds they aren't really wanting rough-and-tumble sex on a regular basis be-cause it is less fulfilling to them at their natural set point.

THE NEEDY LOVER

The Needy Lovers are needy in general, not just in terms of sex. They also may be less affected by the desire curve ups and downs because their need for sex is triggered by a need for stress relief, and there always is enough stress in life to go around. Because the Needy Lover is focused on their own experience, they can unwittingly trigger resentment in their partner, who might feel "used" as a form of stress relief. The Giver (see below) and the Soulful Lover might not mind being used in this way if the needy partner stays present during the lovemaking and isn't just focused on getting his or her way. A Rough-and-Tumble hot sex lover might enjoy this kind of partner because they are presented with a way to dial up the intensity of the sex as sport!

THE GIVER

The Giver gets turned on by giving their partners pleasure. Pertot divides this into two categories, which I have reinterpreted as the true Giver ver-sus the neurotic Giver, who simply gives to get or manipulate. True Giv-ers really and truly get off on other people's pleasure. Their turn-on is literally the partner's turn-on. These people aren't going to mesh with the lovers who have trouble with arousal or generally low levels of spon-taneous or responsive desire. As a result, the Givers will be affected more by plunges in the desire curve of their partners than their own changes. As far as the partner who gives to get, I think that is more a personality issue, probably rooted in the imbalances of their own emotional system's PANIC/GRIEF tonality. They are trying to please partners as a way of manipulation and may be getting off by being martyrs, which is neither fun nor sexy.

THE ANXIOUS LOVER

The Anxious Lover can become so incapacitated by performance anxiety that their self-consciousness can squash their own spontaneous and even responsive sexual desire. This style may be more of a hindrance for men since in general they are expected to initiate sex and perform. The Anxious Lover can experience a big boost in confidence from NRE, which often has the power to temporarily override self-consciousness and anxious feelings, especially in the context of a clearly exuberant partner. As the NRE bump declines, the Anxious Lover feels the loss acutely and may go into self-doubt, worry, or self-consciousness. This lover often has an imbalance in the PANIC/GRIEF system, which predisposes him or her to self-doubt and worry.

THE LOW SEX DRIVER

The Low Sex Drivers typically have a low baseline of desire, regardless of their circumstances. Some may never experience sexual desire or pleasure because they are so blocked in the LUST system. Others may even border on being asexual (people who truly do not want sex, period). NRE may have the impetus to bump up the appetite of the Low Sex Driver, if indeed he/she is capable of accessing sexual desire. If the Low Sex Driver gets into a long-term relationship with an individual with a high sex drive (like the Explorer, see below) and the Explorer partner doesn't mind initiating sex, the responsive sex drive in the Low Sex Driver might be sufficient to keep the sex life alive. Otherwise, this kind of person is a tough match for any other erotic fingerprint except of course another Low Sex Driver.

THE EXPLORER

The Explorer is just like it sounds — someone who is unconstrained by norms and is not only willing to explore sexuality in all sorts of ways but often requires the intensity of the journey itself. They LUST for novelty. The Explorer is simply someone who enjoys tons of new sex activities as PLAY and experimentation. Sexual Explorers can range from the toe dipper to the major full-tilt arctic adventurer. In general, Explorers are not so affected by drops in the desire curve as they are inventive and in general willing to find new ways to turn themselves and others on. They may not mesh well with the Soulful Lovers who need to have soft, gentle, and predictable sex. One important point to consider in relation to Explorers: we have tended to pathologize people in this category as being sensation seekers, and some experts attribute this behavior to deficits in the dopa mine system or some kind of trauma that drives their desire for S & M, for instance. For the record, clinical research has not borne out the notion that kinky people are kinky because of such traumas, although that is typically what laypeople tend to think. Even in popular literature, such as in *Fifty Shades of Grey*, the S & M habits of the protagonist are portrayed as rooted in a history of abuse. I simply believe that these thrill-seekers have a particularly intense SEEKING system, coupled with high LUST. As you will see when we take a look at the lessons from extraordinary lovers, they can teach us a lot about our own capacity for pleasure and what we might find when we go beyond our comfort zones.

Our erotic fingerprints can change over time, particularly if our sexual style is impacted by an imbalance in the core emotions (such as in the case of too much anxiety, as just discussed) rather than reflecting an actual sexual preference, per se. Conceivably, the Needy Lover might become increasingly secure over time and become more attuned to Giver- or Explorer-type energy. Or the Low Sex Driver might find access to a higher baseline sex drive as his or her basement emotional systems rebalance. And conversely, a person's EF may change in response to changes in the other direction; as imbalances show up in the core emotions, an EF might reflect a change where an Explorer whose SEEKING system flattens out a bit might become more of Soulful Lover. Bear in mind that no one EF is intrinsically better or healthier than another; the key here is *vive la différence*.

As you consider your own erotic fingerprint, keep in mind that these are flexible categories and you may find yourself in more than one, depending on your mood or current situation. What's most important, however, is not only honoring where you are at any given point in time but also respecting your partner's fingerprint preferences. Keep in mind too, that fingerprint propensities are malleable, with some people's being more flexible than others. Key to all of this is understanding how your erotic fingerprint intersects with that of your partner. Understanding where you differ, and where you overlap, can provide some good fuel to keep LUST alive.

Navigating Different Erotic Fingerprints: Ella and Louis

Ella, a twenty-nine-year-old accountant and mother of one, is a Soulful Lover with low spontaneous desire. She is married to Louis, a moody artist and sexual Explorer with very high spontaneous desire. When they first met and fell in love, their NRE made Ella's erotic fingerprint much more flexible, so the two seemed quite in tune with each other sexually. However, the NRE wore off, especially after the birth of their daughter and Ella's return to work. As the demands of juggling motherhood and work kick in, Ella's desire begins to dissolve and eventually disappear. She simply doesn't want to have sex anymore and even starts to worry that what turns Louis on is "too kinky." Ella is at her core a Soulful Lover, so Louis's Explorer energy outside of the throes of NRE feels like just too much.

Ella is preoccupied with work and raising their three-year-old daughter, Jillian, and is coming to believe that something is wrong with her husband since he wants to have sex all of the time, and he often wants it to be different.

She wonders if he is some kind of sex addict, but then she backs down and says, "When we first got together, I've got to say I liked how much Louis was into sex. I felt like he really loved and wanted me. I enjoyed experimenting sexually but now I feel like it's just become a big pain in the ass. Like he doesn't want to grow up. He likes to play guitar, and work on his art, and although his gallery is finally making some money, I am still the one who is always worrying about everything, the bills, whether Jillian is being taken care of, whether the roof is leaking. We bought this two-family home, and we live on the first floor, so now we have the responsibility of being landlords, and it mostly falls on me."

Louis disagrees and says in response, "You are always complaining, Ella. No matter what. We have a great life. Jillian is in preschool all day; your accounting practice is doing great and my gallery has taken off. You are no fun anymore. None. All you do is go over the checklist in your head and make demands that I do this or fix that. And you don't acknowledge all of what I do for you and Jillian and the house. You have become such a drag. You were so much fun when we met. And so hot to trot. What the hell happened?"

Both are angry and disappointed and having trouble navigating the building resentments toward the other. Together we worked through the bio/psycho/social steps, trying various tools from bhandas to Kegels to turn on Ella's LUST system, as well as to quiet down Louis's SEEKING system and activate more of his CARE system. It is amazing that working with the bhandas and Kegels can help modulate both overactive as well as underactive sexual energy by helping balance the autonomic nervous system. One tool that helped Ella and Louis tremendously was partner yoga, which brought in the PLAY system in a nonthreatening way for Ella and helped satisfy her need for connection as a Soulful Lover while stimulating Louis's desire for sensual touching and connection. But the most transformational tool we used together in therapy was one that helped Ella and Louis reframe their power struggle using a novel perspective — one that helped them see the dance they were doing in terms of the masculine and feminine. This is what I call the four-quadrant model of the masculine and feminine.

Sometimes emotional imbalances within relationships or disconnects between two people can be addressed by reimagining gender roles. Such an approach helped Ella and Louis to see their masculine and feminine roles more flexibly. I learned this approach from a brilliant teacher, physician, and author, Rudy Ballantine MD. We tend to think of feminine behavior as "relational," involving nurture and taking CARE of others, which Rudy calls the *feminine passive*. And we tend to think of masculine as the propensity to go out and hunt something — to provide, to protect, to rule, to control, to own, which Rudy calls the *masculine active*.

Rudy introduced me to two other quadrants of masculine and feminine — the *masculine passive* and the *feminine active*. The *masculine passive* penetrates a situation with awareness, insight, and understanding, and without rushing into action. The *masculine passive* is energy that we want to cultivate through reflection, meditation, yoga, or therapy. We therapists call that type of self-awareness "the observing ego" and try to cultivate that capacity in clients through our work together.

Feminine active is the energy that gives birth to something new in a way that is expulsive and potentially without consideration of how the new will impact the old. Rudy likened the energy of the feminine active to the goddess Shakti, the cosmic force of creation and change. Similar to when a woman is about to give birth, this process will naturally take over, and happen inevitably (if nothing gets in the way).

When *feminine active* energy arises in a relationship, a danger can be posed to the status quo. And status quo is the province of the *masculine active* — to possess, to own, to protect.

Men and women alike can tap into all four of these roles. Not only can we become more fully formed beings and learn to be more responsive to our partner's different aspects, we naturally become more whole and complete people ourselves. This flexibility enables us to integrate all kinds of energies, bringing other parts of self into the fold of who we are. This approach also allows us to continually renegotiate the premises of our relationships as we grow, incorporating this growth as a sustainable way of relating. Instead of a relationship breaking down when one or the other person makes a change, we give ourselves space for each partner to intentionally cultivate the underdeveloped parts of self that the other partner may have in abundance.

Ella is stuck in the *masculine active* and *feminine passive* roles. She is trying to work and provide, to keep things under control and orderly (*masculine active)* and take CARE of home and family (*feminine passive*). Louis, on the other hand, is majoring in *feminine active* energy — he is trying to create, to change things up, give birth to new stuff in and out of the bedroom, and otherwise challenge Ella's attempts to maintain control over their universe. One way to think about *feminine active* is total SEEKING plus LUST equals birth of something new. And Louis certainly has a whole lot of SEEKING and LUST energy, also very high levels of PLAY, which has him show up like a bit of a Peter Pan, all of which is deeply disturbing to Ella. They are having a massive power struggle, one that is playing out across the pillars of their lives, although the original reason they sought help was the sexual issues.

Ella is trying to keep things even and is stressed constantly that her husband is not on the same page. Louis is becoming increasingly resistant and digging his heels in deeper to rebel. He feels controlled and limited by Ella's anxiety and general anhedonia. This couple is heading for big trouble, especially if Louis goes full-blast Shakti and does something impulsive, like seek sex elsewhere. If we look at the onset of affairs in a marriage, it can often be conceived of as rising up of the *feminine active* energy to spill out unconsciously — giving birth to a new sexual relationship without consideration of the potential destruction of the commitment to the original partner.

This model of the four quadrants of the masculine and feminine gives us a way to conceptualize the dance we do in relationship with self and other. Ideally, as individuals, we can flexibly move between those quadrants as needed in a way that works for us. Ella can embrace her *masculine active* as needed to provide and organize. She can move into *feminine passive* when she needs to nurture and to strengthen her relationships (think also how this maps onto the CARE system). What is underdeveloped in Ella is her ability to engage her *masculine passive* — the ability to witness how she is out of balance herself (too much anxiety — think overactive PANIC/GRIEF system) without rushing in to try to control her anxiety from the outside by attempting to control Louis. Also, Ella could use a big dose of cultivating her own *feminine active* (think ramping up PLAY here through increasing her SEEKING) and going for her own pleasures, requiring that she might have to figure out what they might be. At the root, Ella is anhedonic, and the resistance to explore her husband's high LUST, high PLAY, and high *feminine active energy* is not helping her. She is essentially overfunctioning for Louis by hogging up all of the *masculine active* and *feminine passive* territories and not letting herself explore her other quadrants.

Once Ella and Louis have this model, they become more aware of not only how the imbalances in their emotional basements are playing out, but how they can intentionally cultivate a better balance overall. Both Ella and Louis turn some of their attention (SEEKING) to develop more of the ability to simply witness themselves and the dance they do together (here they are cultivating the *masculine passive,* or "observing," energy). Ella learns to engage SEEKING plus PLAY plus LUST to engage her own *feminine active* energy — to put attention on her own creativity and pleasures. Once Louis senses this shift, he steps up to the plate and attunes more to taking CARE of some of the household worries that Ella had been shouldering (ramping up his *feminine passive,* or nurturing, energies), and simultaneously ramps up his own *masculine active* (taking charge of responsibilities). Once Louis no longer has the monopoly on the SEEKING, PLAY, and LUST energies, and Ella no longer overfunctions in general by taking too much CARE of everything and everyone except herself, things between them become more balanced.

Ella learns to unleash her own Shakti energy in belly dance class. She has always wanted to learn how to be more embodied and seductive and this activity awakens her playful erotic energy, and Louis loves seeing her be in this energy. In response, Louis then makes sure his brother can come over weekly to play with their daughter while he and Ella create more time and place in their schedules for their own grown-up playdates. Ella and Louis are a great example of the importance of learning flexibility when it comes to staying connected to each other and to themselves. By tapping into their operational intelligence and using sex as the conduit, they are not only able to resuscitate their relationship but also heal their respective emotional imbalances — all on the road to pleasure. Ella and Louis are a passionate example of two people who were willing to look beyond their defenses and prescribed roles to discover an amazing degree of satisfying pleasure — a place where they became much bigger to themselves than they ever thought possible.

Whether your journey to pleasure is solo or with someone, you now have some powerful tools that can help you reimagine your own erotic potential.

Enhancing our capacity for sexual pleasure involves expanding the definition of sex to include a broader meaning of the erotic, one that includes that which "enlivens" us. When I talk to clients, I explain that by awakening our appetite for life (via intentionally engaging our SEEK-ING and PLAY systems) such that we get turned on by life itself—by being present and exploring ourselves, each other, and the world with "new eyes" and new enthusiasm, our erotic potential expands. When we turn ourselves on in a bigger way outside the bedroom by living more fully and freely, the energy we unleash can find its way back into the bedroom and fund more LUST plus PLAY with our partners and ourselves.

And reciprocally, by rebooting our sexual pleasure, we set in motion a cascade of beneficial neurochemicals that can trickle down and help restore the balance of our core emotional systems in a dynamic positive feedback loop that continues to lift the spirits and enliven the loins. Pleasure breeds enthusiasm and enthusiasm encourages the very behaviors and results that yield yet more reasons to be exuberant.

In the next chapter, you will learn about some other daring individuals whose journeys led them to discover that their pleasure and enjoyment in sex did not end in midlife, but instead extends for as long as they want. I call this state of ongoing pleasure "sexual potential"—it's a promise that sex, like any and all pleasures, has the capacity to continue, evolve, and adapt to you and your own desires. Ultimately, this potential is realized through harnessing the power of healthy hedonism—and goes way beyond reanimating our erotic lives. Cultivating the practice of healthy hedonism provides fuel for actualizing the potential for a long life worth living. So how do we get on this path of healthy hedonism? Well, you're on it! Just keep playing with the tools, stay in touch with your brain and your body, and a life full of pleasure is yours.

Good Sex Versus Great Sex:
Embracing Your Sexual Potential

The Journeys of Extraordinary Lovers

With your tools to resuscitate your pleasure more at your fingertips, you no doubt are much closer to fully embracing your own hedonic pathway. And perhaps because of this new self-knowledge, you may now appreciate some of my favorite women — those who I consider to be extraordinary lovers because of the way they have pushed the boundaries of their own sexuality in order to explore their widest sexual potential. I have been lucky enough to have this group of women participate in my research; they have helped me further understand the neuroscience of orgasm and explore the many dimensions that make up sexual pleasure. Witnessing their amazing transformations and their sexual journeys confirmed one of the central hypotheses of my work: anyone has the capacity to become an extraordinary lover if they engage their brains and bodies, harnessing their full potential to experience pleasure.

These women volunteered to be part of my research because they were keenly interested in understanding the significance of their own sexuality and felt that others could benefit from their donating their own orgasms to science. But what I learned first and foremost from the ladies of the lab is that their respective paths toward sexual expansion reflected way more than sex. Indeed, just like all my patients over the years, the energy, challenges, issues, and questions that drove these women reflected both their sexuality and their emotional systems. None of these women started out completely comfortable and confident in their sexuality, but they did develop a greater sense of ease and pleasure. Indeed, the journeys that led the women to the lab were ones of personal growth, healing, and transformation, and they embody one of the most central points of this book: our relationship with our sexuality offers us a keen window into our relationship with pleasure in general, and beneath that, the workings of the emotional brain. For these women, unleashing their own sexual potential came about through SEEKING a better understanding of the key role that pleasures of all kinds, including sexual, play in the process of healing and how enlivening their lives in general can naturally spark better sex.

My research participants varied in age and background: a twenty-four-year-old single teacher who was exploring becoming a personal coach, a fifty-eight-year-old divorced woman with four grown children, a forty-seven-year-old Japanese woman who works at a nonprofit, a thirty-three-year-old married actress, and a forty-two-year-old single real estate broker, among others. Some had experienced trauma and sexual abuse. Others emerged from years of religious indoctrination where they were taught that any kind of sexual desire or pleasure is unacceptable and shameful. One woman used to suffer from body dysmorphia, in which she would look at herself in the mirror and be convinced that she was thirty pounds heavier than she really was.

For all of these variations in their backgrounds and starting places, they all have evolved into women who embrace their sexuality and erotic selves.

From Convent School to Sexual Liberation: Lena

Meet Lena, who, at seventy-seven years of age, decided to donate her orgasms to science. Looking at Lena, one would never guess her age. She is a slim, attractive, conservatively dressed woman. In advance of the scanning date, I had instructed her to dress comfortably, and since it is summer, she dons a long A-line sand-colored linen dress. Her earth-tone canvas espadrilles are sensibly low-heeled. One could imagine a woman like Lena always being the mistress of her sexual universe — in fact a mistress of all realms of her life. Poised, articulate, and soft-spoken with a charming Italian accent, she reminds me a bit of a toned-down present-day Sophia Loren, dark hair streaked elegantly with gray, great bone structure, petite but still curvy. Lena seems so self-assured and confident that one would think she was this way across all realms of her life — in and out of the bedroom.

And yet during the preinterview, I learn that Lena has had a rough ride. Born in a small town in Italy, she lost both parents at an early age and was sent away by her aunt to live at a Catholic boarding school — essentially a convent school — at nine years old. She says that her life really didn't start until she got divorced from a highly regarded surgeon, who was essentially a bully. After thirty-two years, she finally gathered up the courage to leave him once the last of her four kids left the nest, and she's never looked back. She enrolled in school, got her law degree, and set out on what she calls a "healing journey" that included taking charge of her sexuality.

"My husband had absolutely no patience with me, my wants and needs, sexually or otherwise. As a doctor, he had knowledge about the body, but he didn't seem interested in helping me learn to have sex. It was my job to satisfy him. To give him the orgasm he wanted. I was in service of his sexuality. I don't think I really ever liked sex with him."

She continued, "When I left my marriage, I made a decision to do whatever it took to build a life. And it was very important to me that I embrace my own sexuality since it was obviously so repressed. This journey has literally taken me a few decades. I went back to school, found a place to live, and then started studying everything — beyond the subjects I had to do for my degree. I made this my passion, my adventure, my mission."

Lena's story embodies so much about how making a conscious decision to prioritize your sexuality can bring joy, health, relationships, and yes — pleasure in all of its many forms. Lena's profound realization that she was sexually repressed, and how her husband reinforced this way of thinking, was like the seed that sprouted her out of that old life. She was hungry to grow, to master life in and out of the bedroom. Lena had to take a big risk to leave a marriage that did not welcome her as a complete and expressed social and sexual being. This huge risk to blow up her life and her marriage was what she needed to break out of the orbit of her repressed sexuality and comforts of the domestic patriarchal life. It was a huge risk for her to go out of her comfort zone and choose to see pleasure in general and her own sexuality pleasure specifically as an important priority. Indeed, sexual potential comes with and from growth and as a development of self.

As the years passed, Lena forged the foundations for a new solo life. She moved to Manhattan, set up a new law practice, and accrued a circle of kindred spirits — both men and women — who shared her passion for growth, including in the sexual realm. These friends formed the matrix of a satisfying social life with a core group who became a kind of family. One of these friends had heard of my research and suggested Lena check out our lab. When she phoned, we connected immediately. She was fascinated by the science and eager to help me fill in the "gaps in the literature" to penetrate the mysteries of the orgasmic brain.

Lena arrived at the Rutgers Brain Imaging Center on a steamy hot July day with her friend Tom (a friend with benefits, she explained) and soon surprised herself (and me too) by having two "magnificent" orgasms in the scanner, no easy feat even for those significantly younger — one orgasm from masturbating, the other from having her clitoris manipulated by Tom.

All extraordinary lovers make their sexuality — and the pleasure of it — a priority in their lives. They don't count orgasms or worry about their performance. They don't measure their experience against anyone's expectations. These qualities of openness, exploration, a turning away from constraining norms (which often attach feelings of shame to sex) are embodied by these Explorers.

A Gap Year for a Grownup: Mary's Excellent Adventure

Extraordinary lovers come in all shapes and sizes, from all sorts of backgrounds and motivations. Meet Mary, an Englishwoman who volunteered for my study as part of a "gap year" she was taking from her life back in the UK. Mary was only in her late forties, but she'd married young, had children right away, and now they were out on their own. She and her husband, Roger, partners in business too, were now empty nesters. Although this juncture can trip up many couples, Mary decided to take this time in her life by storm: she participated in yoga retreats, human potential programs, and felt committed to exploring — inside of herself and the world around her.

She had been a late bloomer, not having her first period until she was almost seventeen, and then got married and had her first child by the time she was twenty-one years old. She'd been raised in a household where her parents slept in separate beds and no one discussed sex — she didn't even know what it was or what it entailed.

Once she was married, she had intercourse with her husband as if it were any other activity — like cleaning the kitchen or making dinner. She didn't expect much from sex. It felt good but wasn't all that compelling. It became part of her routine, something she did because it was something more or less she was supposed to. Her husband seemed to like it well enough, and she was so engaged with work and raising kids that she didn't stop to contemplate what she might be missing.

As time wore on, however, and her children got older, went off to school and then university, and then into their own lives, Mary realized that she had not created any dimension to her life. She didn't know herself well, had little sense of the interior of herself — her thoughts and feelings. She wasn't depressed exactly, but she was "a bit like a shell," as she shared with me. She was curious about what might lie beyond the life she was so accustomed to, what might unfold for her if she shook things up and ventured out into the world.

When she first stepped outside of her small house on the outskirts of London, she took a yoga class. Then she took a painting class. She began to feel her body in new ways. She began to see the world around her in vivid colors. It was as if she'd been literally turned on for the first time. She explained to me that these sensual activities seemed to trigger memories: she'd experience "whiffs" of sensory memories from her early childhood — climbing fences, making mud pies, watching birds fly. These images carried potent feelings of delight that she began to summon and look for again as she began to do more with her days. They were in essence positive, visceral associations from her childhood that had been stored in her midlevel mind and were being rekindled by new experiences. Mary was enlivening the pleasure body by accessing these delicious embodied sensed memories.

One new step gave rise to the next, and Mary began blooming. She and Roger surprised themselves by having long talks into the wee hours about the trajectory of their lives. These talks were compelling. They hadn't engaged this way since early in their relationship. She and Roger realized that while they were quite successful in going through the motions of their well-oiled marital and family life, and had done exceptionally well in launching the family, they had forgotten that they, themselves, were actually quite different, separate people who had become a bit lost to each other. Mary took more risks to share what she was discovering about herself on the yoga mat. One big realization was that she had all of this sexual energy that was unleashing as she advanced in her practice. She felt it in her body. She brought it home to share. She and Roger began to enjoy sex more than ever. And almost paradoxically, now that their sex life had reignited, actually bigger and juicier now than ever, Mary was in touch with a deep hunger to travel the world and experience herself separate from Roger and the family. She wanted to take what she never had as a young person — a gap year — because she had gone directly from school to marriage to making a family. Mary wanted to roam.

And roam she did. Different cities, different friends, even different continents. And strangely enough, Roger was always happy to get a text, a call, a photo, when she sent them, but he didn't require much in the way of long-distance maintenance. He would say — "Go have your experience. Have the most fun and adventure you can, and then bring it all home to me when you are ready." He held down the fort and managed their business while Mary did things such as donate her orgasm to science. Mary and Roger had discovered one of the main ingredients for a relationship with ongoing sexual (and relational) potential. They were secure enough to allow each other space to grow, individuate, and love in a way that promotes both freedom and deep connection. And this is the arc that Mary had brought with her into my lab.

From Sexual Trauma to Erotic Transcendence: Sylvie

Sylvie was an accomplished violinist who had traveled the world professionally for close to twenty-five years. She was a truly unique performer who graced the stages of the most prestigious venues imaginable as she accompanied superstar groups in need of a gorgeous and gorgeously talented soloist who could rip to shreds a violin the way only master guitarists are known to do with their instruments. At age forty she decided abruptly that she was done with playing music when her violin coach, who had become her manager, died suddenly of a heart attack. His death brought Sylvie to a complete standstill. Simon had been her best friend and the only real constant in her life. In fact, Simon was the only one who knew that her previous violin coach had, over time, been sexually inappropriate with her until the abuse became outright sexual molestation when she was in her early teens.

When the abuse happened, Sylvie had told no one. She just kept making excuses for why she didn't want to go to practice. First it was that her belly hurt. Then she had headaches that wouldn't go away. Her parents took her to doctor after doctor who could find nothing wrong. In those days, sexual abuse of children was not part of the cultural consciousness, so no one suspected. And Sylvie didn't volunteer any information. Finally, she came up with a strategy and told her parents that she no longer wanted to study the violin and had simply been too afraid to tell them. This was horrendously disappointing to her family as it was apparent to all that she was exquisitely gifted and somewhat of a prodigy already. But ultimately, they were relieved when Sylvie's symptoms went away and life returned to normal.

Six months later, her dad was transferred to a new location and the family moved. When Sylvie expressed interest the following year in returning to violin lessons (after meeting a girl at school who happened to be studying as well), the parents were thrilled. No one wondered why she all of a sudden became willing to study again, but the good news was that her new teacher was incredibly impressed with Sylvie's skill and she blossomed under his kind tutelage. This teacher was Simon.

Life progressed, and Sylvie thrived. She seemed to be unscathed by her experience. She dated, but clearly her real love affair was with her violin. By a twist of fate, when the other kids were going off the college, Sylvie ended up being booked by a big rock band that leaned heavily on violins. First, she worked with them in the studio. That went well. Then she was asked to go out on tour and basically never turned back. This was her dream come true. She was a rock star with a violin and a fabulous manager who she could trust, who had her back, who reveled in her success.

There were some lovely guys she hooked up with here and there. A few were what she called her frequent flyers. She loved them but didn't feel like she ever was in love. She preferred it this way. Nothing serious. The boys in the band looked out for her. She had fun. She had friends. She wasn't looking to settle down. But when Simon died, she fell apart. She came home, heartbroken, and without a plan.

Simon's death hit everyone hard. He was that special. Simon's older brother contacted her shortly after the funeral. Their cousin was coming into town. His name was Jeff and he was buying a small recording studio in the city. Could Sylvie show him around?

She did more than take him on a tour of the city. Sylvie and Jeff fell in love, and the strongest element of their relationship began with their ability to listen to each other's life story. For the first time, Sylvie was able to be perfectly candid about everything that had happened to her. She also shared the loving moments of her past relationships. This raw honesty enabled Sylvie to be truly open and vulnerable with Jeff, a rawness that spilled over in abundance into their sexual relationship.

Ten years later, Jeff and Sylvie have melded into a power couple. Jeff not only could deal with Sylvie's history of sexual abuse, her "unattached" sexual adventures on the road, but embraced all of her, including her sexually inquisitive nature. They are not afraid to dive into the scariest and most revealing places in themselves and share these details openly and joyfully with each other. They understand how tolerating feelings, especially those that are uncomfortable, is key to it all. They like to explore together and consciously play with the healing power of embracing and unfolding all of their sexual histories together. In becoming comfortable with the uncomfortable, Jeff and Sylvie have been able to forge a magnificent marriage of two very sexual people, exemplifying the incredible power of a pleasurable connection.

Lessons to Live By

Extraordinary lovers share qualities that have been explored in research spearheaded by the Canadian sexologist Peggy Kleinplatz, PhD. Kleinplatz is known for groundbreaking research into how many of our ideas about sex are based on outdated understanding of sexual mores and behaviors. Kleinplatz's research delved into certain types of sexual attitudes and behaviors that have in the past been defined or categorized as pathologic. It was not so long ago that homosexual sex was regarded as abnormal or perverted, for instance. Kleinplatz has pushed against these criteria, suggesting that sexual behavior exists on an enormous continuum and that all of us can actually learn from these "extraordinary lovers," as she refers to them. In several studies, she zeroed in on people who enjoy S & M and found that these lovers tend to be just more interested in sex than the average person. And as already mentioned, they do not have more psychopathology (mental illness, history of trauma or sexual abuse, as previously assumed) than the more "vanilla" (more traditional in the bedroom) type of individuals.

In fact, according to Kleinplatz, the vast majority of problems that bring people into sex therapy stem from what she calls the "North American sex script" that centers on having heterosexual intercourse with orgasms in all the right places, meaning that women should be experiencing orgasms reliably through sexual intercourse, which is actually not the case. Even with additional clitoral stimulation, less than half of women (43 percent) report experiencing orgasm through intercourse 75 percent of the time. In other words, our cultural view of sexuality is narrow, limiting, and performance-oriented, favoring what does not appear to come naturally (pun intended). Along with the other unrealistic expectations we may have about sex, we also expect passionate love to be perpetual and that NRE will last forever. As we've seen, this only sets us up for huge disappointment once we habituate to the relationship. And then we go even a step further: we pathologize ourselves and each other for having "low sexual desire" when in fact it is simply that after NRE wears off, our spontaneous sexual desire returns to baseline. Yet we still have responsive sexual desire lying beneath the surface, waiting to light up if we should give ourselves the time and space to prioritize pleasure and the erotic.

By studying and analyzing these Explorers, Kleinplatz identified a number of characteristics they share, which she enumerated into ten "lessons from the edge." While my ladies of the lab may or may not practice some S & M, they certainly all push the boundaries of what is typical, and they all embody the expansive attitude of erotic pleasure as described by Kleinplatz.

Inspired by my own research and that of Kleinplatz, I have gleaned seven lessons from my own research and work with clients. These lessons apply to all of us who want to leave anhedonia behind and truly embrace our sexual potential.

So what can we learn from extraordinary lovers?

- *Do not judge your erotic self or the erotic experience.* Practice radical self-acceptance. Learn to love your body, exactly as it is. This is one of the biggest lessons, mentioned by nearly all of my participants. They also become curious about their own sexuality and went about exploring what turned them on. Learn to embrace your unique erotic fingerprint — whatever it is. Now that you know the difference between spontaneous and responsive desire, now that you know where you are on your own desire curve, let yourself be exactly as you are in the moment. And let the moment be exactly as it is. Sex is our willingness to be sexual beings, however that shows up. Remember first and foremost that good sex is about being present.
- *Tune in.* Shift your focus inward to listen closely to what you want and what your body yearns for. What are your fantasies? How do you like to be touched? Why not explore all areas of your body that can give you pleasure? And as Beverly Whipple recommends, become keenly aware of what pleases you across

the senses beyond touch — don't forget about sounds and tastes. Are you interested in perhaps being more active when you tend to be receptive? More receptive when you're usually more active? Making subtle shifts in your habitual roles may reveal new ways that you can be turned on. Paying attention to sensations is key for pleasurable sex. If your mind wanders and starts to get into "spectatoring" mode — becoming goal-directed or self-conscious — simply notice that without judgment, letting those thoughts be exactly as they are while you bring your attention back to the senses.

- *Be patient — about getting turned on.* When you want to have intercourse, for example, don't begin until you and/or your partner are sufficiently aroused. Allow the sex to unfold without rushing into it. Although this advice may seem simplistic, it's hugely important to experiencing the pleasure of sex. Slow down and savor the sensations. Let them build. Enjoy the journey without concern about the destination.

- *Stay connected to your partner.* You now have a number of tools to use with your partner — to manage defenses, be an attentive and active listener, and be open to differences in erotic fingerprints or desire. Respect these differences and you will feel more connected. Often the best way to connect is actually going beyond words. Simply do what NRE lovers spend tons of time doing — eye gazing. Look into your partner's eyes and breathe with your partner while sitting silently. See the person in front of you, the being you fell in love with. Spoon your partner and hold them and synchronize your breath to synchronize your nervous systems. This actually works. We are like tuning forks and go into "cardiac" entrainment with lovers (and even our pets) when we settle into the connection. Good sex is connected sex.

- *Take risks.* We often feel hesitant to speak up with partners about parts of ourselves that we think they will judge or worry that if we tell them how we truly feel we will hurt them. We tend to play it safe when in doubt. But another way to look at this is that there is a risk to not taking risks. If we don't explore some of the scarier places with our partners, if we don't explore the corners of our erotic selves, we tend to shut down and stagnate. And stagnation, itself, is dangerous to relationships. Sexual potential unfolds when we bring all of ourselves into the mix. We are always, always shifting and changing and growing. Taking the risk to reveal how these changes impact us, our thoughts, our fears, our feelings, even our fantasies tends to revitalize the partnership.

- *Prioritize pleasure.* Allow sex to play a larger role in your life. Your work with your seven core emotions has paved the way for more keen awareness and insight into how and why pleasure is so important to your life, so allow sex to play a larger role. Make time for sex, expand your notion of what sex is, nurture it, and explore it. It's a journey without an end.

- *Tolerate emotions and embrace the transformative nature of sex.* Because of the blend of emotional and physical drivers of sex, any type of sexual experience or activity has the capacity to stir up all kinds of emotions. One of the most important lessons for good sex and also good relationships in general is to learn how to more fully tolerate our feelings, other people's feelings, and our feelings about other people's feelings. And sometimes the most challenging feelings to tolerate, believe it or not, are intense feelings of pleasure — which for some can feel scarily out of control. When we can learn to simply allow the feelings to be as they are, stay present to ourselves and to each other, the experiences we can have with and through sex can be truly healing and can revitalize our mind, body, and spirit. It is a tangible form of connection to others, a source of immune-boosting energy, and a vast reservoir for pleasure.

These lessons or takeaways offer an invitation to understand and explore yourself and your lover in a whole new dimension of sexual pleasure.

GOOD SEX TOOL: TOUCH PLUS IMAGERY

Remember, neurons that fire together wire together. We can turn up the volume on our genital sensations if we lay down and strengthen those pathways over and over.

This exercise offers you a way to increase your ability to access sensations in your genitals, which will then make it easier to access sexual pleasure. Based on my research, I came up with this exercise after studying the difference between imagined touch and actual physical touch of the genitals.

1. Find a comfortable place where you're not going to be disturbed. Wear comfortable clothes that allow an all-access-pass to your private parts. Put on some nice music and perhaps light a candle. Remember this is time to simply experience your sensations — the intention is not to orgasm.

2. If you're a woman, begin by rhythmically tapping/stroking your clitoris. Concentrate on how your fingers feel as they experience the sensations of touch as you touch

yourself — and then widen your sensory awareness to also include how your clitoris feels receiving the touch.

3. If you happen to have a penis, you can rhythmically tap/ stroke stimulate any place on your penis and likewise concentrate on how your fingers feel as they experience the sensations of touch as you touch yourself — and then widen your sensory awareness to also include how your genitals feel receiving the touch.

4. As you rhythmically tap or stroke genitals, simply register the good or pleasant feelings; this is not intended to be erotic.

5. After about five minutes of tapping, rest a minute or two and notice any sensations that linger post-touch. We tend to not pay keen attention to the full range of our sensations — how they register or ramp up or ramp down. Really tuning into the subtlest of sensations as they build up or release is a good practice to tune into our ability to register sensations.

6. Now, it's time to tune into your imagination. For the next minute or two **just think** about touching your genitals in the same exact way you just did in the first part of the exercise. Tune into the experience — and don't worry if you don't seem to actually "feel" sensations from the genitals by just thinking about them. Focus on the imagined experience.

7. Continue by interspersing rounds of actual touch stimulation with rounds of imagined stimulation and simply pay attention to all of your sensations. The key here is repetition. The more you go back and forth between rounds of touch and rounds of imagined touch, the

more you will prime the power of imagination to access sensations.

Again, this exercise is not meant to lead to an orgasm here or even turn you on. It's designed to teach you how to focus on experiencing sensations from the body both from touching and then imagining touch. You can also do the same with your nipple (whether you are a man or woman), as my research has shown that the nipple also paves a pathway to the place where genital sensations land! You can also practice touching any part of your body (lips, neck, inner thighs, etc.) that you might experience as pleasurable and sensual.

GOOD SEX TOOL: SENSATE FOCUS: HEALTHY HEDONISM VERSION

Sensate focus exercises were created by Masters and Johnson as a treatment for people who are experiencing sexual problems—most often due to their being too self-conscious, anxious, performance-driven and goal-directed to allow nature to take its course in the bedroom. The point is to get people out of their heads and back into the experience of being connected to their sensations and their partners—and getting out of the habit of evaluating their own sexual "performance." Masters and Johnson called this "spectatoring": when we are too busy watching ourselves to see if penises are going to get hard or stay hard or orgasms are going to happen for us or our partners. Sensate focus is all about being mindful of our sensations, rather than focusing on how to "have sex." In fact, in the first stages of sensate focus, it is suggested that you abstain from sex altogether, starting with simply taking turns touching and being touched, at first staying away from the genitals or any sexual "behaviors" and gradually allowing the sensory exploration to expand over time.

There are lots of wonderful resources on the web about sensate focus, and many people have revised and added versions of it. For our purposes we're going to keep it very simple: the point of sensate focus is to get back into your own sensations rather than to focus on providing sensations or pleasure to your partner. And this is a critical point. We want to get back to what feels good to us with and through touching.

One of the things I've noticed as a therapist is that when I assign homework to clients, they often end up not doing it — not because they're trying to sabotage their treatment or want to stay stuck. I think it's because people have this feeling that homework is something they should do, which ends up where they're not really in touch with their wanting to do it. So what I recommend instead is offering my clients — and now you — the basics, and then let you invent what you think would be fun.

1. Decide with your partner when and how you would like to explore sensations. Think of it as playtime in the sandbox. Decide who will go first and establish some boundaries and requests. For example, you might agree that you are going to focus on starting with any body part that is not a genital/breast. You might wish to wear some clothing so that you don't get sidetracked by naked bodies. Make sure that it is clothing that you can feel comfortable in and you can reach arms and legs and heads and shoulders and toes even.

2. Whoever is going to be the first to explore sensation might start by thinking of the imagined genital stimulation exercise as a way of accessing their own imagination. Then the person who is experiencing the sensation simply touches the partner — any part of the body that

you've agreed is okay — and you explore simply the sensations of touch for you, not for them.

3. You might think of using coconut oil as a lubricant for your hands, or whipped cream — anything that would feel good.

4. Tune into the sensations you are having as you touch your partner. Explore his or her body with your fingertips, your lips, your tongue. Concentrate on your own pleasurable sensations. You can experiment with your breathing and working with your pelvic floor to tune into your sensual and sexual energies. (See "Good Sex Tool: Mula Bhandas," page 150.)

     Get more daring with each iteration.

5. After each of you has had your turn being pleasured, take some time to talk about your experience. What was going on in your mind? What was going on in your body? What was going on in your emotions? Share each other's experience and talk about what you would like to try going forward and what you would like to explore in sensation play — let yourself imagine new games to play. Next time only wear a towel or a sarong. Agree in advance to increasing the range of body parts and activities with the caveat that it is play, not production. Rinse, reinvent, and repeat!

Sexual Potential: Your New Frontier

There's a reason Lena, Mary, and Sylvie have become my heroes. Lena, who is almost eighty years old and is a great-grandmother, has weathered and also enjoyed a long, productive life thus far. I believe that one of the reasons for this spirited, vital longevity is her relationship to her own sexuality. Near the end of our work together, I asked her what she might want to share with other women/people on their journey, and she said,

> The most important thing is to get rid of the shame — everything opens up and sex is about being open. I still feel the shame now and then — even a bit of shame about thinking I could be with a woman because you understand how wrong I was taught that would be. But I just let myself deal with it. It's just an old feeling. And I would say, learn to love your body, learn to love yourself, learn to feel like being sexual is good for you. For all of us.

Lena is not only an extraordinary lover but also embodies the notion of sexual potential, which sees the maturation of our sexuality as the "highest mental, emotional, physical, and spiritual level to which we can aspire sexually."

Mary's quest not just for novelty but for personal growth is ultimately the source for her own sexual potential, showing us again how any infusion of energy, any area of growth, flows back into our sexuality and our continued capacity for pleasure. She has provided us a wonderful example of how being separate from our spouses through cultivating our own interests and experiences can supercharge our connections and empower our partnerships for long-term sexual potential.

And Sylvie, who — despite the odds against her due to sexual trauma — not only explored the world on her own but was able to learn to trust an intimate partnership that did not pathologize her sexual experiences and her sexual nature. Sylvie's relationship became a huge part of her healing journey and has taken her to great places of joy and sexual alchemy.

Currently, we have only one model of romantic relationship, and it is founded on the predominance of genital stimulation and intercourse in the context of hot and heavy romantic love. The notion that great sex is the domain of the young who are in hot and steamy passionate love reinforces this limited understanding of sexuality over time. Why would we expect our youth-obsessed culture to teach people anything about the benefits of sexual maturity as a road to bliss? We tend to think that once you get to a certain age, you go into "sexual retirement" and leave the glories of sex to young people.

And yet Lena and others suggest a different experience and a more satisfying journey. Individuals and couples who learn about sexual potential, who see the opportunity to move beyond power struggles, blame, and shame and lean into their fear and anxiety, can often find their way to sexual potential on their own. In fact, it is precisely the ability to lean into the uncomfortable feelings — to tolerate them, feel them fully, acknowledge them, allow them, and risk sharing them with our partners — that ultimately enables our transformation. Being able to tolerate emotional intensity is one of the most important prerequisites for emotional and sexual maturity. Then, and only then, can we confront feelings of disillusionment; dig into letting go of dependency fantasies; and deal with the real partners in front of us, rather than expectations of who the partner "should be." Disillusionment in our sex lives and our relationships is the starting point for the quest, rather than the point at which we should abandon the "sinking" ship and seek new waters. How cool is that? What a different frame!

Being able to recognize, experience, and tolerate the feelings we have been taught to shut down — the oversocialization that truncates our ability to have the full range of emotional experiences — grief, sadness, fear, anger, felt and honored and acknowledged all the way through — is what enlivens us and allows us to tolerate and embrace and be present to the joys as well. Those who manifest their sexual potential intentionally cultivate the ability to be playful, curious, and creative. When we learn how to soothe our defensive systems through self-CARE, connect with our social engagement systems and each other, harness the power of the SEEKING and PLAY systems, LUST for life becomes accessible.

That is what emotional regulation is at its best — not asking us to limit or push down the feelings but to lean into them, while at the same time recognizing that rushing into action or reaction is not operationally intelligent. The Gestalt therapists used to say, "Lose your mind and come to your senses." Hot seats are like that: you go through the sadness to the anger, and then even deeper, beneath and below that, to the attachment and back to the joy and laughter when you follow the thread of emotions to their roots.

Risk knowing more about yourself and your partner every day. Your self-awareness and ability to take responsibility for yourself rather than blame your partner will facilitate personal insight and relationship growth. Each day we shift, grow, and change such that being with a partner becomes more of a habit than anything. Pay attention to how you are new each day and how your partner shifts. Be willing to risk uncomfortable truth telling and shaking up the status quo. Rethink how you do your everyday habits, your habitual interactions, and really sit down with new eyes for each other. One practice I recommend to clients is to end each day with listening to each other's high and low points from the day — and climbing into their experience with new ears and new eyes.

And as much as connection with our partners is critical, developing our sexual potential hinges on cultivating the ability to be both a part of and apart from a relationship — what we therapists have called "differentiation" as whole, complete human beings — whole and growing, rather than broken people who lean on each other for completeness. It is about getting increasingly comfortable in your own skin and risking being your authentic self while connecting deeply and transformationally with your partner.

Mature relationships are based more on wanting the connection and all that goes with it—rather than "needing" it to be "complete." Our well-being doesn't hinge on how any one particular external resource or relationship looks in the moment. Paradoxically, we can go way deeper with someone when we know we are whole and emotionally separate. And going deeper and wider is key to actualizing our sexual potential, an ongoing, ever-changing dynamic that can unfold across the lifespan.

So are we after good sex or great sex?

Curiously enough, in yet another paradox of our overly analytical minds, seeking great sex outright is not the answer. Dr. Beverly Whipple, a true boundary-breaker in the field of human sexuality, teaches that when we focus on seeking great sex, we get into a kind of striving mindset. We become goal-directed. We start evaluating the experience rather than being in the present moment. *Is this going to be as good as last week? Is this better than yesterday?*

The negative side effects of the process of evaluation become glaringly evident in people who struggle to "achieve" an orgasm. As I am fond of saying, a watched orgasm never boils. We tend to more easily *experience* orgasm when we relax into sensations and let the orgasm find us. If it does, great. If it doesn't, why not fully enjoy the experience exactly as it is? Some people who regularly and reliably orgasm don't find the experience particularly satisfying, while others find their sexuality immensely satisfying and pleasurable regardless of whether they orgasm or not.

Why are these demarcations about the quality of sex so important? By widening our expectations about what sex is and getting past any goalposts for what we deem "good" or "great," we actually give ourselves the opportunity to experience so much more pleasure and so much more of ourselves. Indeed, that's the underlying truth about sexual potential: relieving ourselves of expectations makes our ability to experience sexual pleasure limitless. It's an attitude, a mindset. There is no restriction from functioning, age, or situation. Actualizing our sexual potential is a practice that can keep us enlivened, sexy, healthy, happy, and connected. Actualizing our sexual potential can keep us turned on to living.

A Final Note

As I put the final touches on the book, I am flooded with a tangy sweet mix of emotions. Big joy is present in bolus doses. Could I have ever believed that the twenty-two-year-old kid I once was, the girl who felt irrevocably broken in the wake of her first panic attack, could look back on her younger self from this vantage point? Having forged a mostly joyful and deeply meaningful life from teaching what I, myself, have needed to know, I feel blessed. I am passing along the lessons received from my own teachers — the yoga instructors, psychotherapists, mindfulness mavens, clinical supervisors, clients, patients, my kids, my husband, other researchers, and other writers who have indelibly pressed their lessons, delivered via different pathways, into the matrix that has become me. My own spin comes mostly from weaving this into a tapestry, influenced both by my view from the basement of the brain **and** the top of the mind — with utmost desire (SEEKING) to know how to guide ourselves more from conscious commitments than by emotional weather. I have cultivated the fine art of being both an anxious soul and a calm, confident, courageous, **PLAY**ful creator (**my own recipe**). And I have been incredibly fortunate along the way to have intrinsically been more curious (**SEEKING**) than afraid (although the FEAR level is not trivial).

As this book comes to a close, I also grieve. There never seems to be enough time to totally complete anything that is truly important. Whether it is a dissertation, a scientific study, a manuscript, a book, parenting our children, or loving another human being — we are always, always faced with the imperfection and incompleteness of actual real life. This is the source of our deepest regrets. What we could've, should've, would've done. But beneath that, it is also the source of our biggest joys and satisfaction. We **CARE** enough to want to create a completely perfect conclusion to what we truly care about.

One of the big highlights in winding up this book: Life is full catastrophe. Think Zorba the Greek: We are born, we die. We celebrate, we mourn. People get injured, people get sick, and no one gets out alive. None of this ultimately ends well, as my dear husband often reflects (to cheer me up) when, from time to time, we get mired in the muddy bottom of despair. No matter how hard we try to rearrange the deck chairs of the Titanic, the ship goes down, as my wild and woolly Radical Honesty trainer, Big Bad Brad liked to say over a big fat shot of bourbon. And yes, this might sound depressing on first glance, but being in touch with the awesome realties of both pain and pleasure is what allows us to live and love more fully. As Osho, the groovy conscious guru once *supposedly* said, "The only hope is no hope!" Translated into operational intelligence, what I take that to mean is that once we allow ourselves to be present to what is — to accept (to the extent what we can) what is immediately in front of us, we can release our expectations (which are truly the source of emotions when they are violated — both for better or worse) and be here. And *here* is where it all is. The willingness to be present to whatever is here for the moment is one of the best definitions of happiness I have ever heard. (Thank you, wise soul and Buddhist nun, Pema Chodron — one of my best teachers from afar).

So, wrapping up this baby of a book?

I hope that you feel newly encouraged and empowered to treat yourself, your emotions, your life as "Operationally Intelligent" as possible. That you discover through these stories and tools and insights that you can move into your own pleasure pathway. And that you rediscover and realize that wherever you are, wherever you've been, and wherever you are going, that sex — joyful, erotic, fun, satisfying sex — is your birthright.

So enjoy — good sex really does matter!

Acknowledgments

This book comes as the culmination of many decades of searching for tools and knowledge that could be employed to calm the anxious beast of my own nervous system. First and foremost, I want to acknowledge my family of orientation — my parents, who bequeathed me the genetic predisposition for tremendous curiosity (SEEKING), a good amount of intellectual capacity, and alas, a PANIC/GRIEF system armed and ready for activation. They also provided a home environment that encouraged communication and emotional expression. I believe this fostered my desire to become a psychotherapist, a profession that continues to give me great joy.

The long gestation period of this book (at least twice as long as that of an elephant!) has been a labor of love. The project began when, as a newly minted PhD in 2014, I reached out to Billie Fitzpatrick to explore the possibility of writing about the lessons I had learned from the ladies of my lab — the participants of my orgasm brain studies. Billie thought there was something more to this story and introduced me to the brilliant agent, Yfat Reiss Gendell, who immediately had a vision for an even bigger book—one that embraced the ongoing challenge I faced in my practice as a psychotherapist, which we have come to call "the pleasure crisis." This pleasure crisis is evident in clients stuck in anxiety, depression, and a general malaise, blocking their ability to savor their lives. Working with Billie and Yfat on this project has been a joy: they are a dream team and to them I will always be grateful. I am proud to say that the book we have given birth to has already been useful to my clients with whom I have shared bits and pieces during the course of writing.

And this journey would have never launched without the encouragement of my mentor, dear friend, and sex-science rock star, Dr. Beverly Whipple. I met Beverly years ago at a training sponsored by the American Association of Sexuality Educators Counselors and Therapists (AASECT) while completing my certification as a sex therapist. Beverly invited me to join a research project she was doing with Dr. Barry Komisaruk (with whom, coincidentally, I had taken graduate courses decades before) and the next thing I knew, I was a fifty-year-old graduate student embarking on a PhD in sex neuroscience under Barry's tutelage. Barry and Beverly have paved a path that I am humbled and honored to follow.

I want to also acknowledge my editors at HMH—Deb Brody and Olivia Bartz. Deb came up with the brilliant title at our very first meeting. She has shown unwavering enthusiasm for the project. And Olivia's great insights and edits helped me refine my ideas.

Lastly, I want to acknowledge my fabulous husband, John, who is also my best friend, partner in crime, father of my children, and grandfather of my grandchildren. Who knew when we met as teenagers that we were heading for such a long, strange, adventurous, loving, and delicious trip?

Notes

Introduction

page

ix *I have presented my pilot data to the Society for Neuroscience:* Barry R. Komisaruk, Nan Wise, Eleni Frangos, Wendy Birbano, and Kachina Allen. "*An fMRI Video Animation Time Course Analysis of Brain Regions Activated during Self-Stimulation to Orgasm in Women*." Abstract. Society for Neuroscience (2011). Program number 495.03.

xiv *As Bob Dylan once said:* Bob Dylan. "Subterranean Homesick Blues" (1965). Columbia Records catalogue number 43242.

xv *Pursuing this giant hunch, I dived into a seven-year PhD program:* Nan Wise. "Genital Stimulation, Imagery, and Orgasm in Women: An fMRI Analysis." PhD diss., Rutgers University, Newark, 2014.

1. The Theft of Pleasure

4 *I am certainly not alone in confronting this massive pain epidemic:* Christopher M. Jones et al. "Vital Signs: Demographic and Substance Use Trends Among Heroin Users — United States, 2002–2013," *Morbidity and Mortality Weekly Report* 64, no. 26 (2015): 719-25 and Yuri P. Springer et al. "Notes from the Field: Fentanyl Drug Submissions — United States, 2010–2017," *Morbidity and Mortality Weekly Report* 68, no 2 (2019): 41–43.

5 *A 2017* New York Times *article reported:* Katharine Q. Seelye. "As Overdose Deaths Pile Up, a Medical Examiner Quits the Morgue," *New York Times,* October 7, 2017.

https://www.nytimes.com/2017/10/07/us/drug-overdose-medical-examiner
.html.

This drug use — both prescriptive and illegal: William C. Reeves et al. "Mental Illness
Surveillance Among Adults in the United States," *Morbidity and Mortality Weekly Report 60,* no 3 (2011): 1–32.

7   *In part, many of us have inherited a vulnerability to anhedonia:* Martin Seligman has acknowledged both our evolutionarily inherited propensity for worry and our capacity
for cultivating optimism and resilience. In a recent book, he talks about the mind as a
tongue that is always looking for a broken tooth.

> What happened to the brain that believed "It is a nice day today; I'm sure it will be
> a nice day tomorrow"? This brain was crushed by tomorrow's ice. The brain that
> believed "Today may seem like a nice day, but tomorrow comes the trouble" survived
> and passed its genes down to us. Paranoia — to say nothing of depression, anxiety,
> and anger — has major survival advantages in a world that is actually full of danger,
> loss, and injustice.

Martin E. P. Seligman. *The Hope Circuit: A Psychologist's Journey from Helplessness to
Optimism* (London: Hachette UK, 2018): Kindle edition, 209.

10   *Clinically speaking,* anhedonia: A prominent clinical feature of depression is anhedonia, or the relative inability to experience pleasure from previously pleasurable activities. Paul A. Keedwell et al. "The Neural Correlates of Anhedonia in Major Depressive Disorder," *Biological Psychiatry* 58, no. 11 (2005): 843–53.

11   *In many ways, the brain-body is in a constant battle to stay in balance and regulate:* Dr.
Hans Selye, an endocrinologist, pioneered early studies of stress as a response to
aversive events and formulated the concept of the General Adaptation Syndrome.
Later in his career, he expanded the notion of stress to include "eustress" or beneficial
responses to stressors. He posited that stressors that cannot be resolved or actively
coped with would lead to persistent distress that could result in physical and psychological symptoms, while stressors that facilitate effective coping and enhance functioning, and are important to growth and development — hence, the term "eu," or
"good," stress. Hans Selye. "Confusion and controversy in the stress field," *Journal of
Human Stress* 1, no. 2 (1975): 37–44.

12   *Each waking moment of our day asks our built-in stress response to adapt to the environment*: Francisco Mora et al. "Stress, Neurotransmitters, Corticosterone and Body–
Brain Integration," *Brain Research* 1476 (2012): 71–85; Elizabeth N. Holly and Klaus
A. Miczek. "Ventral Tegmental Area Dopamine Revisited: Effects of Acute and Repeated Stress," *Psychopharmacology* 233, no. 2 (2016): 163–86.
*Some people are particularly vulnerable to maladaptive stress responses, including those
who are genetically prone to addiction:* David Ball. "Addiction Science and Its Genetics."
Addiction 103, no. 3 (2008): 360–67.

13   *Historically, we've had a love-hate relationship with sex and pleasure*: Anna Blackburn

Wittman and L. Lewis Wall. "The Evolutionary Origins of Obstructed Labor: Biped-alism, Encephalization, and the Human Obstetric Dilemma," *Obstetrical & Gynecolog-ical Survey* 62, no. 11 (2007): 739–48.

14 *Since that time, thinkers, psychologists, and other scientists have more or less kept this di-vision between hedonia and eudaimonia:* Morten L. Kringelbach and Kent C. Berridge. "Towards a Functional Neuroanatomy of Pleasure and Happiness," *Trends in Cogni-tive Sciences* 13, no. 11 (2009): 479–87.

16 *Our society has had a long, challenging relationship with pleasure:* Jean M. Twenge, Ryne A. Sherman, and Brooke E. Wells. "Declines in Sexual Frequency among American Adults, 1989–2014." *Archives of Sexual Behavior* 46, no. 8 (2017): 2389-2401; Jean M. Twenge, Ryne A. Sherman, and Brooke E. Wells. "Sexual Inactivity During Young Adulthood Is More Common Among U.S. Millennials and iGen: Age, Period, and Cohort Effects on Having No Sexual Partners After Age 18." *Archives of Sexual Behav-ior* 46, no. 2 (2017): 433–40.

   Our culture has deep roots in a Calvinism that associates pleasure (especially sexual or sensual) with shame and places a higher value on stoicism: Eric Luis Uhlmann et al. "Im-plicit Puritanism in American Moral Cognition," *Journal of Experimental Social Psy-chology* 47, no. 2 (2011): 312–20.

17 *In distinguishing between happiness and pleasure, psychologist Dr. Margaret Paul:* Mar-garet Paul. "The Difference Between Happiness and Pleasure," *Huffington Post,* June 14, 2015. https://www.huffpost.com/entry/the-difference-between-happiness-and-pleasure_n_7053946.

2. The Sexual Route to Understanding Pleasure

25 *My early results showed clearly that for all the involvement of the body in the production and experience of an orgasm:* Barry R. Komisaruk, Nan Wise, Eleni Frangos, and Kachina Allen. "An fMRI Time-Course Analysis of Brain Regions Activated during Self-Stimulation to Orgasm in Women." Abstract. Society for Neuroscience (2010). Program number 285.06.

26 *One of the original goals of my research was to fill a huge gap in the scientific literature:* Barry R. Komisaruk et al. "Women's Clitoris, Vagina, and Cervix Mapped on the Sensory Cortex: fMRI evidence." *The Journal of Sexual Medicine* 8, no. 10 (2011): 2822–30.

   Since the neurosurgeon Wilder Penfield originally mapped the somatosensory cortex in the 1950s: When the pioneering cartographers of the brain explored the wiring of the sensory and motor cortices during brain surgery done to treat epilepsy (Wilder Pen-field and Theodore Rasmussen. "The Cerebral Cortex of Man: A Clinical Study of Localization of Function," *The Journal of the American Medical Association* 144, no. 16 [1950]: 1412), the electrical stimulation of the surface of the brain in the region of the paracentral lobule — what we have come to call the genital sensory cortex — resulted in patients' stating that they were aware of sensations in the penis (no female patients were studied), but the patients did not report the sensations to be of an erotic nature. Whether this was simply because they were embarrassed to report being sexually aroused; or whether the context of having the skull open and stimulated by electrodes in an operating room was just not conducive to experiencing sexual sensation; or whether erotic experience involves other, supplementary sensory processing regions — is not entirely clear.

Following the publication of our paper, "Women's Clitoris, Vagina, and Cervix Mapped on the Sensory Cortex: fMRI evidence," other researchers started to integrate our findings into their studies and call attention to the need to further investigate sex differences in the brain's representation of the body. See Paula M. Di Noto et al. "The Hermunculus: What Is Known about the Representation of the Female Body in the Brain?" *Cerebral Cortex* 23, no. 5 (2012): 1005–13.

My research focused on what is happening in the brain during genital stimulation and orgasm: Wise. "Genital Stimulation, Imagery, and Orgasm: An fMRI Analysis." PhD diss., Rutgers University, Newark, 2014.

27 *My initial experiments clearly supported the notion that the "mind" is the most powerful sexual organ of all*: Nan Wise, Eleni Frangos, and Barry R. Komisaruk. "Tactile Imagery Somatotopically Activates Genital Sensory Homunculus: fMRI Evidence," Abstract. Society for Neuroscience (2010). Program number 800.6.

The scans from the experiment showed activations of the paracentral lobule: Nan Wise, Eleni Frangos, and Barry R. Komisaruk. "Activation of Sensory Cortex by Imagined Genital Stimulation: An fMRI Analysis," *Socioaffective Neuroscience & Psychology* 6, no. 1 (2016): 31481.

My studies indicate the brain is so widely and strongly activated by orgasm: Nan Wise, Eleni Frangos, and Barry R. Komisaruk. "Brain Activity Unique to Orgasm in Women: An fMRI Analysis." *The Journal of Sexual Medicine* 14, no. 11 (2017): 1380–91.

28 *In these studies, I also wanted to understand more about female sexual response:* The only other research lab that has investigated brain correlates of orgasm (Janniko R. Georgiadis et al. "Regional Cerebral Blood Flow Changes Associated with Clitorally Induced Orgasm in Healthy Women," *European Journal of Neuroscience* 24, no. 11 [2006]: 3305–16) found deactivations in frontal cortical regions using Positron Emission Tomography (PET) scans, while our previous studies indicated overall frontal activation associated with orgasm. My dissertation sought to resolve this discrepancy in the literature.

29 *This interdependent relationship between pleasure and pain is part of our survival network*: As noted by Morten L. Kringelbach et al. in *The Pleasure Center: Trust Your Animal Instincts* (New York: Oxford University Press, 2009): Kindle edition, 21–22,

> And not only are our brains and bodies hardwired to experience the sensations of pain and pleasure, but also to learn from — and be in turn modified and shaped by

— both painful and pleasurable experiences. Rather than ignore or fight these drives toward pleasure, we might consider how important this information is toward guiding us to towards the pleasures of eating when hungry, drinking when thirsty, having sex when horny, pursuing social and emotional connection when lonely, enjoying the warm feelings of caring for self and others, and last but not least, pursuing the pleasures of play that fuel feelings of social joy.

While the pain system has its own dedicated transmitter, wired to pick up damage to the body: Masanori Otsuka and Mitsuhiko Yanagisawa. "Pain and Neurotransmitters," *Cellular and Molecular Neurobiology* 10, no. 3 (1990): 293–302.

31   *In other words, there is utility to both pain and pleasure:* Siri Leknes and Irene Tracey. "A Common Neurobiology for Pain and Pleasure," *Nature Reviews / Neuroscience* 9, no. 4 (2008): 314–20.

32   *What I began to realize as I delved more deeply into the neuroscience research:* The core emotional systems to which I refer here come from the pioneering work of neuroscientist Jaak Panksepp, who mapped out seven wired-in core emotional operating systems that are explored in detail in chapter 3. Jaak Panksepp, *Affective Neuroscience: The Foundations of Human and Animal Emotions* (New York: Oxford University Press, 2004).

3. The Core Emotions in the Brain's Basement

39   *My insight into the brain's processing systems originated in part from my specific work with an amazing neuroscientist:* Panksepp, *Affective Neuroscience;* Charles Darwin, *The Expression of the Emotions in Man and Animals* (New York: Oxford University Press, 2009).

Panksepp's groundbreaking experimental investigations, which led to his identifying seven core wired-in emotional systems underlying animal and human emotions, adds an important dimension in understanding the roots of our emotions largely unexamined in psychology.

Some believe Panksepp will in time be appreciated as a paradigm shifter taking the work of Darwin forward to advance contemporary psychology's understanding of our core emotions. Kenneth L. Davis, personal communication, 2018.

An excellent source for additional information on the evolutionary approach to emotions and personality can be found in Kenneth L. Davis and Jaak Panksepp's *The Emotional Foundations of Personality: A Neurobiological and Evolutionary Approach* (New York: W. W. Norton & Company, 2018).

40   *But Panksepp's work showed exactly this:* Panksepp, *Affective Neuroscience,* Kindle edition, 1888–89.

In this figure: A. R. Damasio et al. "Subcortical and Cortical Brain Activity during the Feeling of Self-Generated Emotions," *Nature Neuroscience* 3, no. 10: 1049–56.

41   *This table:* Jaak Panksepp. "Cross-Species Affective Neuroscience Decoding of the
     Primal Affective Experiences of Humans and Related Animals," *PLOS ONE* 6, no. 9
     (2011): e21236.
     Panksepp identifies three levels of emotional experience: Panksepp, "Cross-Species Affec-
     tive Neuroscience Decoding," e21236.

42   *These "raw" emotions in the bottom of the brain are fast and are experienced vividly, by
     man or animal:* Jaak Panksepp and Lucy Biven, *The Archaeology of Mind: Neuroevolu-
     tionary Origins of Human Emotions, Norton Series on Interpersonal Neurobiology* (New
     York: W. W. Norton & Company, 2012), Kindle edition.
         *Even human babies born with a rare condition in which the neocortex does not develop
         exhibit these core emotions:* D. Alan Shewmon, Gregory L. Holmes, and Paul A. Byrne.
         "Consciousness in Congenitally Decorticate Children: Developmental Vegetative
         State as Self-Fulfilling Prophecy," *Developmental Medicine and Child Neurology* 41,
         no. 6 (1999): 364–74.
     The next level of emotional experience, the "secondary processes": Panksepp, "Cross-
     Species Affective Neuroscience Decoding," e21236.

43   *And at the top of the brain is the slow, effortful processing:* As Panksepp points out, in
     order for the top-level processes to work effectively, they need to be integrated with
     both the emotions at the core primary level as well as the secondary processes of
     learning from experiences, which are not always conscious. Panksepp, "Cross-Species
     Affective Neuroscience Decoding," e21236.

44   *But anhedonia has created a cleft in this finely designed system:* Panksepp refers to the
     limbic system as the source from which our "impulse for emotionality emerges." In
     this way, he conceptualizes the limbic system as functioning as a "visceral nervous
     system." Panksepp, *Affective Neuroscience,* Kindle edition, 2423–24.
         Animal models that link stress to anhedonia have been proposed. There is empir-
     ical support for the effects of stress to induce anhedonic behaviors in rats. Angela J.
     Grippo et al. "Neuroendocrine and Cytokine Profile of Chronic Mild Stress-Induced
     Anhedonia," *Physiology & Behavior* 84, no. 5 (2005): 697–706.
         The chronic stress anhedonia model has also been extrapolated to explain the
     often-deleterious effects of chronic stress on human physical and mental well-being.
     Stress has been well known to exacerbate anxiety and depression as well as other
     mental and physical illnesses. Recent evidence is even linking stress with tumor de-
     velopment and suppression of the immune system's ability to prevent cancer metas-
     tasis. Mohd Razali Salleh. "Life Event, Stress and Illness." *The Malaysian Journal of
     Medical Sciences* 15, no. 4 (2008): 9–18.

45   *It was Panksepp's research into the significance of these core emotions:* Learning how our
     wired-in mammalian emotional systems give rise to our "raw emotions" gave me in-
     sights as to how psychotherapies that did not deal with these embodied emotions
     could not be effective. Fortunately, affective balance therapies, which recognize and

address the primary process emotions, are becoming increasingly popular. Diana Fosha, Daniel J. Siegel, and Marion F. Solomon, eds. *The Healing Power of Emotion: Affective Neuroscience, Development & Clinical Practice* (New York: W. W. Norton & Company, 2009), Kindle edition.

46   *#1 SEEKING:* Information on the SEEKING system and its role in motivating and energizing the other emotional systems can be found in chapter 8, "SEEKING Systems and Anticipatory States of the Nervous System," Panksepp, *Affective Neuroscience.*

James Olds did the seminal work on how "rats can be made to gratify the drives of hunger, thirst and sex by self-stimulation of their brains with electricity." He went on to say, "It appears that motivation, like sensation, has local centers in the brain." James Olds. "Pleasure Centers in the Brain," *Scientific American* 195, no. 4 (1956): 105.

48   *With anhedonia, there can be many triggers or causes for disruption of the SEEKING system:* Panksepp called this system, "the brain sources of eager anticipation, desire, euphoria, and the quest for everything." He notes that depression and lethargy are often the results "when the SEEKING system is chronically underactive." Panksepp and Biven, *The Archaeology of Mind,* 99.

49   *#2 FEAR:* Information on the FEAR system, which is genetically programmed to prepare animals to perceive and anticipate dangers, can be found in chapter 11: "The Sources of Fear and Anxiety in the Brain." Panksepp highlights the ancestral role FEAR plays, in that many fears do not need to be learned and are in a sense instinctual — such as the fear of pain, and for rats, the smell of cats. Panksepp, *Affective Neuroscience.*

50   *The amygdala, a key player in fast, automatic emotional pathways:* Dominic T. Cheng et al. "Human Amygdala Activity during the Expression of Fear Responses," *Behavioral Neuroscience* 120, no. 6 (2006): 1187–95.
Once conditioned, FEAR learning is set down in the midbrain: In explaining our inherent vulnerability to posttraumatic stress disorders and the potency of fear learning, Panksepp states, "All mammals can be afflicted with PTSD because we all have very similar ancient FEAR systems that can become sensitized and full of trepidation within the cognitive darkness of our core affective consciousness." Panksepp and Biven, *The Archaeology of Mind,* 176.

52   *How does this stress response get so dysregulated and overreactive:* Although short-term release of cortisol mobilizes the fearful animal to flee, excessive amounts of cortisol secreted by the overly stressed and anxious animal (or person) can actually result in damage to the organism's ability to regulate the stress reaction and have negative effects on the brain and visceral organs. As Panksepp notes, "Many resulting stress-induced cascades in the brain and body can contribute to these adverse effects as well. Prolonged high cortisol levels are common in a number of psychiatric syndromes, most especially in depression." Panksepp and Biven, *The Archaeology of Mind,* Kindle edition, 108–109.

53 #3 *RAGE:* Information on the roots of the RAGE system and how it can be easily elicited by frustrating an animal in seeking fulfillment of its needs and its pursuits can be found in chapter 10, "Nature Red in Tooth and Claw: The Neurobiological Sources of Rage and Anger." Panksepp, *Affective Neuroscience*. A further discussion of the distinctions between the raw, "primary process" experience of "rage," the more fully elaborated thought-infused secondary process of "anger," and the highly "incubated" and hard-boiled experience of "hatred" is well covered in Panksepp and Biven, *The Archaeology of Mind*.

What makes RAGE hard to study in humans: On the few occasions that the core RAGE circuits have been electrically stimulated by accident during the course of brain surgery on human patients, it has resulted in intense, aversive experiences on the part of the unfortunate patients. H. E. King. "Psychological Effects of Excitation in the Limbic System." *Electrical Stimulation of the Brain* (1961): 477–86.

55 *I've observed that many people don't feel entitled to feel angry unless they feel they have been wronged or victimized*: This false belief has significant interpersonal consequences and is a common source of relationship distress. Brent J. Atkinson. *Emotional Intelligence in Couples Therapy: Advances from Neurobiology and the Science of Intimate Relationships* (New York: W. W. Norton & Company, 2005).

56 *Aggression is yet another story, with even more twists and turns*: For an exploration of the various types of aggression, see Kenneth E. Moyer. "Kinds of Aggression and Their Physiological Basis." *Communications in Behavioral Biology* 2, no. 2 (1968): 65–87.

57 *As we will examine more fully in chapter 8, there are real differences in the neural circuitry of male and female brains*: The behavioral link between testosterone and aggression, although well established in the animal world, is a controversial topic when examining humans, with conflicting reports depending on many variables. The administration of androgens to biological females seeking to become males (female to male transsexuals) was clearly associated with an increase in aggression proneness, sexual arousability, and spatial ability performance. In contrast, it had a deteriorating effect on verbal fluency tasks. And conversely, the administration of cross-sex hormones to biological males seeking to become females (male to female transsexuals) resulted in decreased aggression, sexual arousability, and spatial task performance. Stephanie H. Van Goozen et al. "Gender Differences in Behaviour: Activating Effects of Cross-Sex Hormones." *Psychoneuroendocrinology* 20, no. 4 (1995): 343–63.

In a study in which testosterone was administered to both males and females, the neural circuits involved in aggression became more responsive to the presentation of angry (but not happy) faces when sensitized by exposure to the administered testosterone. Erno J. Hermans, Nick F. Ramsey, and Jack van Honk. "Exogenous Testosterone Enhances Responsiveness to Social Threat in the Neural Circuitry of Social Aggression in Humans." *Biological Psychiatry* 63, no. 3 (2008): 263–70.

One additional consideration is that behaving aggressively can actually increase levels of testosterone. There is, however, recent evidence that indicates that exogenously administered testosterone will increase aggressive behavior in dominant men. Justin M. Carré et al. "Exogenous Testosterone Rapidly Increases Aggressive Behavior in Dominant and Impulsive Men." *Biological Psychiatry* 82, no. 4 (2017): 249–56.

On another note, although testosterone mediates the sex drive in both males and females, there is some indication that supplementing with too much testosterone in women may actually have a deleterious effect on the sex drive, as it may increase aggression, which in turn limits the potential for sexual interactions. Jill M. Krapf and James A. Simon. "A Sex-Specific Dose-Response Curve for Testosterone: Could Excessive Testosterone Limit Sexual Interaction in Women?" *Menopause* 24, no. 4 (2017): 462–70.

58   *#4 PANIC/GRIEF:* Information on the wiring and function of the PANIC/GRIEF system can be found in chapter 14, "Loneliness and the Social Bond: The Brain Sources of Sorrow and Grief," Panksepp, *Affective Neuroscience.*

This system contributes to protecting our "life-sustaining social bonds": As Panksepp says so eloquently: "At the outset, we are utterly dependent creatures whose survival is founded on the quality of our social bonds — one of the remaining great mysteries, and gifts, of nature." Panksepp, *Affective Neuroscience,* Kindle edition, 9729–30.

Early childhood experiences fundamentally shape the basic tonality of the PANIC/GRIEF system: One of the most robust findings in psychology is the effect of early childhood experiences with caregivers on long-term well-being. For the reader unfamiliar with attachment theory, I highly recommend reviewing John Bowlby's and Mary Ainsworth's extensive writings on it. John Bowlby. *Attachment and Loss: Loss* (New York: Basic Books, 1980) and Inge Bretherton. "The Origins of Attachment Theory: John Bowlby and Mary Ainsworth," *Developmental Psychology* 28, no. 5 (1992): 759–75.

As noted by Panksepp, the first six years of childhood are a vulnerable time for the development of secure bonds with caregivers. Early loss and/or inadequate caregiving can result in "sensitization" of the PANIC/GRIEF system with long-term deleterious effects in terms of high levels of anxiety and depression. Panksepp and Biven. *The Archaeology of Mind,* Kindle edition, 314.

59   *#5 CARE:* Extensive background information about the CARE system can be found in chapter 13, "Love and the Social Bond: The Sources of Nurturance and Maternal Behavior," Panksepp, *Affective Neuroscience.*

Bryan Ferry, the lead singer of the band Roxy Music, once sang, "love is the drug and I need to score": This lyric is from a song written by Bryan Ferry and Andy Mackay of the band Roxy Music, released as the lead single on the album *Siren* in 1975.

60   *The CARE system runs on internal opioids:* Opioid is a modern term used to refer to

any substance that binds with opioid receptors. This includes both natural opiates and synthetic substances. Hugh C. Hemmings and Talmage D. Egan. *Pharmacology and Physiology for Anesthesia: Foundations and Clinical Application* (New York: Elsevier Health Sciences, 2012).

"The physiology of motherhood is the physiology of love," is a quote from Jaak Panksepp, "The Science of Emotions," TEDxRainier, April 5, 2017.

When the CARE system becomes dysregulated, we feel emotional pain: As noted by Panksepp, modest doses of opioids have quick-acting antidepressant effects which have not been clinically employed due to concerns of addiction at higher doses. It would appear that psychic pain can result from either a deficient CARE system or overactive PANIC/GRIEF system, or some combination of both. Panksepp and Biven, *The Archaeology of Mind,* Kindle edition, 348.

62   #6 PLAY: For a detailed discussion of the PLAY system and its role in development, socialization, learning, and joy, refer to chapter 15, "Rough-and-Tumble Play: The Brain Sources of Joy," in Panksepp, *Affective Neuroscience.*

Humans are wired by nature to be neotenous: Panksepp, *Affective Neuroscience,* Kindle edition, 10605–06. Not only do we take a long time to grow up, our frontal lobes are not fully developed until our midtwenties. Elizabeth R. Sowell et al. "In Vivo Evidence for Post-Adolescent Brain Maturation in Frontal and Striatal Regions," *Nature Neuroscience* 2, no. 10 (1999): 859–61.

63   *While there are several kinds of PLAY:* Rough-and-tumble PLAY is so important that the lack of it might be driving the increase in the prevalence of attention deficit hyperactivity disorders. Jaak Panksepp. "Can PLAY Diminish ADHD and Facilitate the Construction of the Social Brain?" *Journal of the Canadian Academy of Child and Adolescent Psychiatry* 16, no. 2 (2007): 57–66.

     And it is even possible to model the benefits of PLAY therapy in rats: Jaak Panksepp, Jeff Burgdorf, Cortney Turner, and Nakia Gordon. "Modeling ADHD-Type Arousal with Unilateral Frontal Cortex Damage in Rats and Beneficial Effects of Play Therapy." *Brain and Cognition* 52, no. 1 (2003): 97–105.

65   #7 LUST: Everything you may have wanted to know about the LUST system (but were afraid to ask) is covered in chapter 12, "The Varieties of Love and Lust: Neural Control of Sexuality," Panksepp, *Affective Neuroscience.*

     And sex is not just about sex. Sexual behavior involves fuzzy and "friendly companionship," which Panksepp deems, "essential for mental health in humans, and probably most other mammals." Panksepp, *Affective Neuroscience,* Kindle edition, 8298–99.

We have tons of data on this that my colleague, mentor, and dear friend Dr. Beverly Whipple: Beverly Whipple. *The Health Benefits of Sexual Expression* (New York: Planned Parenthood Federation of America, 2007).

67   *Our core emotional lives affect us more than we have acknowledged in current psychology:*

Piotr Winkielman and Kent C. Berridge. "Unconscious emotion." *Current Directions in Psychological Science* 13, no. 3 (2004): 120–23.

4. Rebalancing Your SEEKING System: Liking What You Need

74 *Historically, neuroscientists, cognitive psychologists, and other researchers who have studied the brain:* Panksepp notes that the reward/reinforcement centers have been traditionally associated with "pleasure" but are more accurately involved in "foraging, seeking, and positive expectancies," which is the SEEKING system. This system is designed to get us to pay attention and learn from experiences. Satoshi Ikemoto and Jaak Panksepp. "The Role of Nucleus Accumbens Dopamine in Motivated Behavior: A Unifying Interpretation with Special Reference to Reward-Seeking," *Brain Research Reviews* 31, no. 1 (1999): 6–41.

75 *Beginning with the early behaviorists:* B. F. Skinner. "Operant Behavior," *American Psychologist* 18, no. 8 (1963): 503–515.
    What emerged from this line of early experiments was how rewards figure into the way we learn: James Olds and Peter Milner. "Positive Reinforcement Produced by Electrical Stimulation of Septal Area and Other Regions of Rat Brain." *Journal of Comparative and Physiological Psychology* 47, no. 6 (1954): 419–27.
    Other researchers were able to determine that the "reward" system essentially goes flat once learning happens and a signal predicts the "reward" — and consequently the stimuli itself is no longer experienced as rewarding. Jeffrey R. Hollerman and Wolfram Schultz. "Dopamine Neurons Report an Error in the Temporal Prediction of Reward during Learning." *Nature Neuroscience* 1, no. 4 (1998): 304–309; Wolfram Schultz. "Dopamine Reward Prediction Error Coding." *Dialogues in Clinical Neuroscience* 18, no. 1 (2016): 23–32.

76 *Underlying the motivation to obtain pleasure is our brain's prediction or expectation of a pleasurable reward:* Kringelbach and Berridge, "Towards a Functional Neuroanatomy." Lekneś and Tracey, "A Common Neurobiology for Pain and Pleasure."
    Most of this process is enabled by mesolimbic dopamine that operates from the midbrain: Roy A. Wise and Pierre-Paul Rompre. "Brain Dopamine and Reward." *Annual Review of Psychology* 40, no. 1 (1989): 191–225 and John D. Salamone and Mercè Correa. "The Mysterious Motivational Functions of Mesolimbic Dopamine," *Neuron* 76, no. 3 (2012): 470–85.
    When in good working order, the SEEKING system is supposed to function like this: A. Der-Avakian and Athina Markou. "The Neurobiology of Anhedonia and Other Reward-Related Deficits," *Trends in Neurosciences* 35, no. 1 (2012): 68–77.

77 *For years, up through much of the 1980s, scientists thought that the dopamine spikes actually generated or enabled the pleasure from the stimuli:* Kent C. Berridge and Morten

L. Kringelbach. "Neuroscience of Affect: Brain Mechanisms of Pleasure and Displeasure," *Current Opinion in Neurobiology* 23, no. 3 (2013): 294–303.

78   *This relationship between wanting and seeking, the hallmark of the dopaminergic system, is more complicated yet:* Schultz, "Dopamine reward prediction error coding."
However, he and others have pointed out: Schultz, "Dopamine Reward Prediction."
There are two types of dopamine at play in learning that comes from prediction error: Stan B. Floresco et al. "Afferent Modulation of Dopamine Neuron Firing Differentially Regulates Tonic and Phasic Dopamine Transmission." *Nature Neuroscience* 6, no. 9 (2003): 968–73; Wolfram Schultz. "Getting Formal with Dopamine and Reward," *Neuron* 36, no. 2 (2002): 241–63.

79   *However, some people are genetically predisposed to have low levels of tonic dopamine:* Abdalla Bowirrat and Marlene Oscar-Berman. "Relationship between Dopaminergic Neurotransmission, Alcoholism, and Reward Deficiency Syndrome," *American Journal of Medical Genetics Part B: Neuropsychiatric Genetics* 132B, no. 1 (2005): 29–37.

80   *Some aspects of this pleasure cycle are conscious, but most are nonconscious and happen below the level of our awareness:* As Panksepp has noted, our core emotional experiences stem from such an ancient place in our brain/minds — a "phenomenal consciousness" that predates the conscious awareness systems that developed far later in our evolution. Jaak Panksepp. "Neurologizing the Psychology of Affects: How Appraisal-Based Constructivism and Basic Emotion Theory Can Coexist," *Perspectives on Psychological Science* 2, no. 3 (2007): 281–96.
The underlying neurobiology reveals that people with a disrupted SEEKING system are unable to: Der-Avakian and Markou. "The neurobiology of anhedonia and other reward-related deficits."

83   *This loss of spontaneous desire is incredibly common for women and also for some men:* Rosemary Basson. "Using a Different Model for Female Sexual Response to Address Women's Problematic Low Sexual Desire," *Journal of Sex & Marital Therapy* 27, no. 5 (2001): 395-403 and Eric J. Meuleman and Jacques J. van Lankveld. "Hypoactive Sexual Desire Disorder: An Underestimated Condition in Men," *BJU International* 95, no. 3 (2005): 291–96.
Regardless of who is experiencing the LUST fallout: As far as the chemistry of new relationship energy being wild and woolly: Helen E. Fisher et al. "Intense, Passionate, Romantic Love: A Natural Addiction? How the Fields That Investigate Romance and Substance Abuse Can Inform Each Other," *Frontiers in Psychology* 7 (2016): 687.

5. Hot-Tempered and Afraid: Taming Our Defenses

93   *Approximately forty million Americans, about 18 percent of the population, are diagnosed with an anxiety disorder:* Anxiety disorders include generalized anxiety disorder, pho-

bias, obsessive compulsive disorder, posttraumatic stress disorder, and social anxiety disorder. P. S. Wang et al. "Twelve-Month Use of Mental Health Services in the United States: Results from the National Comorbidity Survey Replication," *Archives of General Psychiatry* 62, no. 6 (2005): 629–40.

Our fear response, which is located very near the pain pathway, incorporates the periaqueductal gray (PAG): Cornelius T. Gross and Newton Sabino Canteras. "The Many Paths to Fear," *Nature Reviews Neuroscience* 13, no. 9 (2012): 651–58.

94   *So how does Katie's embedded fear response get untangled from her capacity to orgasm:* Sex educator, pro-sex feminist, and author Betty Dodson has long been a proponent of teaching women to learn how to masturbate. She has published numerous books and created experiential workshops to teach the fine art of self-love. See Betty Dodson, *Liberating Masturbation: A Meditation on Self-love* (New York: Bodysex Designs, 1974); *Selflove & Orgasm* (New York: Betty Dodson, 1983); and *Sex for One: The Joy of Self-Loving* (New York: Harmony Books, 1997).

There has been empirical support of the efficacy of her methods in helping previously anorgasmic women learn to experience orgasm. Pia Struck and Søren Ventegodt. "Clinical Holistic Medicine: Teaching Orgasm for Females with Chronic Anorgasmia Using the Betty Dodson Method," *The Scientific World Journal* 8 (2008): 883–95.

96   *What pushes these new learnings and ultimately transforms her relationship with her own sexuality:* Edward W. Eichel, Joanne De Simone Eichel, and Sheldon Kule. "The Technique of Coital Alignment and Its Relation to Female Orgasmic Response and Simultaneous Orgasm," *Journal of Sex & Marital Therapy* 14, no. 2 (1988): 129–41.

97   *Once you bring your body into an open and relaxed place, calming your emotional system:* Further information as to how neurolinguistic programming can be used in therapy is provided in Juliet Grayson and Brigid Proctor, "Neuro-Linguistic Programming," in Stephen Palmer (Ed.), *Introduction to Counselling and Psychotherapy: The Essential Guide* (London: SAGE Publications, 2000): 159–71.

99   *Very close to the brain-body's FEAR system is the RAGE system:* The reader who seeks further information on the roots and functions of our ancestral RAGE and FEAR systems can refer to chapters 4 and 5 in Panksepp, *The Archaeology of Mind.*

101   *What I immediately pick up on after hearing Kara's history and observing her behavior:* Our hard-earned cognitive insights and desires to regulate our emotions and behaviors can easily dissolve in the wake of the jet stream of our tenacious core emotional habits bubbling up from our emotional basements. Fosha et al., *The Healing Power of Emotion,* Kindle edition, 12.

103   *Ultimately, in order to sustain these positive, affiliative emotions, Kara needs to heighten her SEEKING system and get more turned on by her life:* As Panksepp notes, the SEEKING system is the "granddaddy of all of the emotional systems" and needs to be upregu-

lated in order to boost access to the other emotions. Panksepp, *The Archaeology of Mind*.

An effective therapist engages the client's SEEKING system, and through creating a caring and attuned relationship with the client, allows for a "resonance" that is healing of the client's imbalanced PANIC/GRIEF and other core systems. Panksepp notes that the relationship between the therapist and the client is key in the healing process, which is consistent with the views of Carl Rogers, who viewed the therapist's capacity for empathy as a critical component of effective therapy. Carl R. Rogers. "Empathic: An Unappreciated Way of Being." *The Counseling Psychologist* 5, no. 2 (1975): 2–10.

Ongoing research supports the notion that the quality of the therapeutic relationship is significantly more important than the specific therapeutic intervention used. In other words, a positive therapeutic relationship may be a necessary and sufficient condition for the benefits of psychotherapy regardless of the theoretical approach to the treatment. Michael Lambert and Dean E. Barley. "Research Summary of the Therapeutic Relationship and Psychotherapy Outcome," *Psychotherapy Theory, Research, and Practice* 38, no. 4 (2001): 357.

104 *Dismantling RAGE*: Jaak Panksepp and Margaret R. Zellner. "Towards a Neurobiologically Based Unified Theory of Aggression." *Revue Internationale de Psychologie Sociale* 17 (2004): 37–61.

Let's unpack this neurobiology further: For background information on the hypothalamus and the autonomic nervous system, see Bob Garrett and Gerald Hough, *Brain & Behavior: An Introduction to Behavioral Neuroscience* (Thousand Oaks, CA: Sage Publications, 2017).

105 *If you are like most, you are not a big fan of being enRAGED*: Even animals do not like when their RAGE circuits are stimulated, indicating that they experience it as aversive. See chapter 10 in Panksepp, *Affective Neuroscience*.

Daniel Goleman used the term "amygdala hijacking" in his book *Emotional Intelligence* (New York: Bantam, 2006), referring to work done by Joseph E. LeDoux ("The Amygdala: Contributions to Fear and Stress," in *Seminars in Neuroscience*, vol. 6, no. 4 (Cambridge, MA: Academic Press, 1994): 231–37.

I prefer to refer to this process of being derailed by emotion as limbic hijacking because the amygdala does not act alone — nor, for that matter, does any brain region, but rather in concert with the other structures of what is called the limbic system.

The limbic system, a circuit or brain region involved in emotion, was first proposed in 1937 by James A. Papez. "A Proposed Mechanism of Emotion," *Archives of Neurology & Psychiatry* 38, no. 4, 725–74.

For more information of the evolutionary roots of jealousy-induced anger, see Jaak Panksepp, "The Evolutionary Sources of Jealousy: Cross-Species Approaches to Fundamental Issues," in S. L. Hart and M. Legerstee (Eds.), *Handbook of Jealousy: Theory, Research, and Multidisciplinary Approaches* (Hoboken, NJ: Wiley-Blackwell, 2010): 101–120.

And regarding findings on the heritability of aggression, see Robert R. H. Anholt and Trudy F. C. Mackay, "Genetics of Aggression," *Annual Review of Genetics* 46 (2012): 145–64.

For an interesting perspective on how anger leads us to seek someone to blame, see J. R. Averill, "Ten Questions about Anger That You May Never Have Thought to Ask," in Farzaneh Pahlavan, *Multiple Facets of Anger: Getting Mad Or Restoring Justice?* (Hauppauge, NY: Nova Science Publishers, 2011).

107 *As Panksepp and others have noted, the ability to constructively and productively express anger (what is cognitively layered over the RAGE system) is key to emotional balance:* The regulated expression of anger can serve to increase feelings of empowerment and well-being. Learning how to honestly and productively express anger in therapy can promote better emotional and interpersonal health. Fosha et al., *The Healing Power of Emotion*, Kindle Edition, 11.

There is compelling evidence that either extreme, repressing anger or habitually raging with anger, can have significant deleterious effects on both physical and mental health. Mihaela-Luminiţa Staicu and Mihaela Cuţov. "Anger and Health Risk Behaviors," Journal of Medicine and Life 3, no. 4 (2010): 372–75.

6. CARE, GRIEF, and PLAY: Using Our Affiliative Emotions to Enhance Pleasure

111 *It goes without saying that without CARE:* Extensive background information about the CARE system can be found in chapter 13, "Love and the Social Bond: The Sources of Nurturance and Maternal Behavior." Panksepp, *Affective Neuroscience.*

112 *And sometimes even in the case when parenting has been more than adequate: "Born This Way"* is a single from the album of the same name released by Lady Gaga on February 11, 2011.

Early childhood experiences fundamentally shape the basic tonality of both the CARE and the PANIC/GRIEF systems: Further information on how early childhood experiences affect the tone of the CARE and PANIC/GRIEF systems can be found in chapter 13, "Love and the Social Bond: The Sources of Nurturance and Maternal behavior" and chapter 14, "Loneliness and the Social Bond: The Brain Sources of Sorrow and Grief."

114 *Understanding your attachment style and the tonality of your wired-in defensive systems:* Two popular books on the applications of understanding how attachment styles affect relationship are Amir Levine and Rachel Heller, *Attached: The New Science of Adult Attachment and How It Can Help You Find — and Keep — Love* (New York: Penguin,

2012) and Stan Tatkin, *Wired for Love: How Understanding Your Partner's Brain and Attachment Style Can Help You Defuse Conflict and Build a Secure Relationship* (Oakland, CA: New Harbinger Publications, 2012).

At a neurobiological level, both the giving and the receiving of care is activated by internal opioids: Jaak Panksepp, Eric Nelson, and Steve Siviy. "Brain Opioids and Mother-Infant Social Motivation," *Acta Paediatrica* 83 (1994): 40–46.

115   *It's more accurate to suggest that oxytocin's effects are context dependent:* And it may be more the case that oxytocin is enhancing a sense of trust or confidence rather than warm-and-fuzzy feelings per se. Andreas Meyer-Lindenberg. "Impact of Prosocial Neuropeptides on Human Brain Function," *Progress in Brain Research* 170 (2008): 463–70 and Jennifer A. Bartz et al. "Social Effects of Oxytocin in Humans: Context and Person Matter," *Trends in Cognitive Sciences* 15, no. 7 (2011): 301–9. And as far as my reference to the neurotransmitter dopamine as being the "slutty neurotransmitter": There is widespread support of dopamine playing a big role in reward-seeking behaviors. Óscar Arias-Carrión and Ernst Pöppel. "Dopamine, Learning, and Reward-Seeking Behavior." *Acta Neurobiologiae Experimentalis* 67, no. 4 (2007): 481–88.

When the CARE system becomes dysregulated: It would appear that psychic pain can result from either a deficient CARE system or overactive PANIC/GRIEF system, or some combination of both. Panksepp, *The Archaeology of Mind.*

116   *As you may have experienced, the undesired breakup of an important romantic relationship is often accompanied by signs of withdrawal:* Naomi I. Eisenberger. "The Pain of Social Disconnection: Examining the Shared Neural Underpinnings of Physical and Social Pain," *Nature Reviews Neuroscience* 13, no. 6 (2012): 421–34.

117   *Although Liza feels she's doing the right thing by staying home to take care of her two kids:* Aside from the stress involved in parenting taking its toll on our sex lives, it appears that the hormones oxytocin and prolactin, both of which are implicated in maternal/parenting behaviors, may have an inhibitory effect on testosterone, which may impact libido. Oxytocin appears to mediate the refractory period in men and also be responsible for the post-orgasm glow of both men and women. Panksepp, *Affective Neuroscience,* Kindle edition, 8509–10.

Too much prolactin can negatively impact testosterone levels and sexual functioning in men: Scott I. Zeitlin and Jacob Rajfer. "Hyperprolactinemia and Erectile Dysfunction," *Reviews in Urology* 2, no. 1 (2000): 39–42.

Administering oxytocin to human fathers resulted in lowered testosterone levels, which were associated with more optimal parenting. Omri Weisman, Orna Zagoory-Sharon, and Ruth Feldman. "Oxytocin Administration, Salivary Testosterone, and Father-Infant Social Behavior," *Progress in Neuro-Psychopharmacology and Biological Psychiatry* 49 (2014): 47–52.

118 *I also reassure her that this is very common for new parent couples:* The distinction between active/spontaneous and receptive sexual desire is an important one, originally
made in reference to a new model for female sexual desire. It is important for both
men and women to recognize that it is not uncommon to experience a reduction
in the "active" sexual desire in long-term relationships or after the birth of children.
Rosemary Basson. "Using a Different Model for Female Sexual Response to Address
Women's Problematic Low Sexual Desire."

119 *I know that their therapy will not take much time:* The reference to the habits for relationship success comes from the work of Dr. Brent Atkinson, a pioneer in synthesiz-
ing empirical work done by the Gottman relationship laboratory (see below) with
new findings in affective neuroscience.

Here are a few resources for the lay reader:

John M. Gottman, Julie Schwartz Gottman, and Joan DeClaire. *Ten Lessons to
Transform Your Marriage: America's Love Lab Experts Share Their Strategies for
Strengthening Your Relationship* (New York: Harmony Books, 2007).

Dr. Atkinson has a workbook for couples (*Developing Habits for Relationship Success: A Step-by-Step Guide for Improving Your Relationship,* version 4.6), which can be
obtained directly from his website: https://thecouplesclinic.com/books/.

For those interested in learning more about Dr. Atkinson's pragmatic/experien-
tial approach to therapy:

Brent J. Atkinson. *Emotional Intelligence in Couples Therapy: Advances from Neurobiology and the Science of Intimate Relationships* (New York: W. W. Norton & Company, 2005).

Brent Atkinson et al. "Rewiring Neural States in Couples Therapy: Advances
from Affective Neuroscience." *Journal of Systemic Therapies, Special Issue: Psychotherapy and Neuroscience* 24, no. 3 (2005): 3–16.

120 *She books a weekend at a yoga retreat for herself (alone!):* The exercise I suggest to Liza,
recommended to me by Dr. William Stayton — an incredibly gifted psychologist, sex
therapist, and Baptist minister — involves using *The Joy of Sex* by Alex Comfort (New
York: Simon and Schuster, 2003). Here are some of Dr. Stayton's published works for
the interested reader:

William R. Stayton. "A Theology of Sexual Pleasure," *SIECUS Report* 30, no. 4
(2002): 27–30.

Yolanda Turner and William Stayton. "The Twenty-First Century Challenges to
Sexuality and Religion," *Journal of Religion and Health* 53, no. 2 (2014): 483–97.

121 *Good Sex Tool: Active Listening, part 1:* The concept of active listening was proposed
as an important therapeutic tool by Carl Rogers. Carl Ransom Rogers and Richard
Evans Farson. *Active Listening* (Chicago: Industrial Relations Center of the University
of Chicago, 1957).

Harville Hendrix and others have developed various active listening exercises to enhance communication. Harville Hendrix, Helen LaKelly Hunt, Wade Luquet, and Jon Carlson. "Using the Imago dialogue to deepen couples' therapy." *The Journal of Individual Psychology* 71, no. 3 (2015): 253–72.

124 *In addition, her lack of appetite for anything to nurture herself:* When survivors of the Holocaust suffer from clinical depression, PTSD, or anxiety disorders that interfere with their capacity to parent, it can result in attachment issues in their children.

Harvey A. Barocas and Carol B. Barocas. "Separation-Individuation Conflicts in Children of Holocaust Survivors," *Journal of Contemporary Psychotherapy* 11, no. 1 (1980): 6–14.

It is encouraging, however, to note that most children of holocaust survivors do not manifest psychopathology, which is a testament to the resilience of the survivors and their offspring. Natan P. Kellerman. "Psychopathology in Children of Holocaust Survivors: A Review of the Research Literature." *Israel Journal of Psychiatry and Related Sciences* 38, no. 1 (2001): 36–46.

125 *In order to make her feel more whole, her therapy needs to pump up her social engagement system:* The social engagement system is a concept put forth by Stephen Porges in polyvagal theory that the human nervous system developed the capacity to be impacted by our interactions with others. Soothing positive social interactions encourage optimal operation of our nervous and endocrine systems and can downregulate our reactions to stress. In order for us to develop as healthy individuals, our social engagement systems need to be operating effectively. Stephen W. Porges. "Social Engagement and Attachment," *Annals of the New York Academy of Sciences* 1008, no. 1 (2003): 31–47 and Stephen W. Porges. "The Polyvagal Theory: Phylogenetic Substrates of a Social Nervous System," *International Journal of Psychophysiology* 42, no. 2 (2001): 123–46.

129 *The Wondrous Potential of PLAY*: For a detailed discussion of the PLAY system and its role in development, socialization, learning, and joy, refer to chapter 15, "Rough-and-Tumble Play: The Brain Sources of Joy," in Panksepp, *Affective Neuroscience.*

130 *So, Henry's body doesn't seem to be the issue here. It is his head. He is suffering from a bad case of "spectatoring"*: Masters and Johnson coined the term "spectatoring," or watching/observing oneself during sex, rather than actually being present in the experience. They felt that much of sexual dysfunction stemmed from being too self-conscious in this way. William H. Masters and Virginia E. Johnson. *Human Sexual Inadequacy* (Boston: Little, Brown, 1970).

133 *The bottom line is that play is good for your health:* Joseph A. Doster et al. "Play and Health among a Group of Adult Business Executives," *Social Behavior and Personality: An International Journal* 34, no. 9 (2006): 1071–80; Kathrin Gerling et al. "Ageing

Playfully: Advancing Research on Games for Older Adults beyond Accessibility and Health Benefits," in Proceedings of the *2015 Annual Symposium on Computer-Human Interaction in Play* (2015): 817–20.

7. Operational Intelligence and Creating a New Way to Be

137 *But what actually ends up happening is that we suffer from what's known as the hedonic treadmill:* The term "hedonic treadmill" was coined by Philip Brickman and Donald T. Campbell in 1971. Mortimer H. Appley et al. *Adaptation-Level Theory: A Symposium* (Cambridge, MA: Academic Press, 1971): 287.

We each have a general set point of happiness: David Lykken and Auke Tellegen have done pioneering work in determining the heritability of subjective well-being or happiness. "Happiness Is a Stochastic Phenomenon," *Psychological Science* 7, no. 3 (1996): 186–89. The notion that you can intentionally decide what to do with the genes you inherit and the circumstances was a key ingredient in the learned optimism put forth by Martin E. P. Seligman. *Learned Optimism: How to Change Your Mind and Your Life* (New York: Vintage, 2006).

140 *Creating a New Recipe:* Dr. Milton Erickson was the founder of Ericksonian hypnotherapy. He was a pioneering psychiatrist who was able to effect therapeutic changes in the most challenging of client situations and an important influence on the development of the Neurolinguistic Programming (NLP) conceived by Richard Bandler and John Grinder. Richard Bandler and John Grinder. *Reframing: Neuro-Linguistic Programming and the Transformation of Meaning* (Boulder, CO: Real People Press, 1979).

I completed advanced training as a practitioner in Ericksonian hypnotherapy at the NLP Center in New York in 2002. Milton H. Erickson and Ernest Lawrence Rossi. *Hypnotherapy: An Exploratory Casebook* (New York: Irvington Publishers, 1979).

This permission acts as a powerful suggestion that helps to soften our tensions: I participated in "Clinical Training in Behavioral Medicine" at Harvard Medical School's Mind Body Institute in February and March 1994. It is now known at the Benson-Henry Institute for Mind Body Medicine. Dr. Herbert Benson, its founder, is a pioneer in cardiology and what he calls "remembered wellness," another term for the placebo effect, which is the body's own ability to rebalance and heal. He is the author of a number of books about the relaxation response and behavioral medicine. Herbert Benson and Miriam Z. Klipper. *The Relaxation Response* (New York: Morrow, 1975).

141 *Janet then grounds this new recipe in her body by making a practice audio tape:* I refer to Yogic breath exercises that include Mula Bhanda or "Root Lock," which is the first of

these energy locks that are essential to Kundalini yoga. It is accessed by contracting
the muscles of the center of the perineum and has a positive impact on the nervous,
respiratory, circulatory, endocrine, and energy systems of the body. Sravana Borkataky
Varma. "The Ancient Elusive Serpent in Modern Times: The Practice of Kuṇḍalinī
in Kāmākhyā or The Elusive Serpent," *International Journal of Dharma and Hindu
Studies* 1: 63–85.

*Breath work calms the nervous system, which enables us to access our underlying systems
and experience the feelings themselves*: Pallav Sengupta. "Health Impacts of Yoga and
Pranayama: A State-of-the-Art Review," *International Journal of Preventive Medicine* 3,
no. 7 (2012): 444.

   Richard P. Brown and Patricia L. Gerbarg. "Sudarshan Kriya Yogic Breathing
in the Treatment of Stress, Anxiety, and Depression: Part I — Neurophysiologic
Model," *Journal of Alternative & Complementary Medicine* 11, no. 1 (2005): 189–201
and Varma, "The Ancient Elusive Serpent."

142 *Good Sex Tool: Breath Basics:* During the exhalation phase of breathing, parasympathetic tone is increased as the vagal brake kicks in to slow down the heart's pacemaker.
This promotes a vagal state of calm. By extending the outbreath a bit longer than the
in breath, we can increase parasympathetic tone, which feels good and is good for
you.

   Stephen W. Porges. *The Pocket Guide to the Polyvagal Theory: The Transformative
Power of Feeling Safe* (New York: W. W. Norton & Company, 2017), Kindle edition,
447–48.

144 *From a neuroscience perspective, the excitement of "unpredictability and uncertainty"*:
Hollerman. "Dopamine Neurons Report an Error," 304 and Schultz. "Dopamine Reward Prediction Error Coding," 23.

145 *So what tools do they use individually and as a couple to reboot their pleasure system?:*
Ujjayi, or ocean breath, is a technique used so that you can hear the sounds of your
own breath as you practice yoga. You can also use ujjayi breath sounds as the focus
of meditation. There are a multitude of breath tools as well as yoga postures that are
effective in restoring a sense of calm and well-being necessary for the ability to experience pleasure. Brown, "Sudarshan Kriya Yogic Breathing," 189–201 and Caroline
Smith et al. "A Randomised Comparative Trial of Yoga and Relaxation to Reduce
Stress and Anxiety," *Complementary Therapies in Medicine* 15, no. 2 (2007): 77–83.

147 *Good Sex Tool: Active Listening, part 2:* Dr. Harville Hendrix and his wife, Helen, are
internationally known couples' therapists and the founders of Imago therapy. I have
been influenced by their work on the importance of listening to and validating our
partners' feelings. Harville Hendrix. *Getting the Love You Want: A Guide for Couples*
(New York: St. Martin's Griffin, 2007).

150 *Good Sex Tool: Mula Bhandas:* Mula Bhanda is the first of three energy locks essen-

tial to Kundalini yoga. It is accessed by contracting the muscles of the center of the perineum and it positively impacts the nervous, respiratory, circulatory, endocrine, and energy systems of the body. Varma, "The Ancient Elusive Serpent."

Mula Bhanda practice, like Kegel exercises, which are similar, will strengthen the floor of the pelvis and improve blood flow to the genitals.

The strengthening of the pelvic floor in women is associated with improved sexual functioning. Lior Lowenstein et al. "Can Stronger Pelvic Muscle Floor Improve Sexual Function?" *International Urogynecology Journal* 21, no. 5 (2010): 553–56; Kristen M. Carpenter, Kristen Williams, and Brett Worly. "Treating Women's Orgasmic Difficulties." *The Wiley Handbook of Sex Therapy* (2017): 57–71

Strengthening the pelvic floor with Kegels has been shown to be an effective treatment for erectile dysfunction in men and lifelong premature ejaculation. Grace Dorey et al. "Pelvic Floor Exercises for Erectile Dysfunction," *BJU International* 96, no. 4 (2005): 595–97.

151 *Good Sex Tool: Yoga:* Yoga has been shown to increase improve sexual functioning in women. Vikas Dhikav et al. "Yoga in Female Sexual Functions," *The Journal of Sexual Medicine* 7, no. 2 (2010): 964–70; Lori A. Brotto, Lisa Mehak, and Cassandra Kit. "Yoga and Sexual Functioning: A Review," *Journal of Sex & Marital Therapy* 35, no. 5 (2009): 378–90; Lori A. Brotto, Michael Krychman, and Pamela Jacobson. "Eastern Approaches for Enhancing Women's Sexuality: Mindfulness, Acupuncture, and Yoga (CME)," *The Journal of Sexual Medicine* 5, no. 12 (2008): 2741–48.

Yoga has been shown to increase testosterone levels in both men and women· R. S. Minvaleev et al. "Postural Influences on the Hormone Level in Healthy Subjects: I. The Cobra Posture and Steroid Hormones," *Human Physiology* 30, no. 4 (2004): 452–56.

153 *Early on in my career, I was fortunate enough to work with "big, bad" Brad Blanton:* Brad is a psychologist, Gestalt therapist, author, workshop leader, and founder of Radical Honesty International. Brad Blanton. *Radical Honesty: How to Transform Your Life by Telling the Truth* (Stanley, VA: Sparrowhawk Pub., 2005). I participated in his intensive residential workshops in practicing radical honesty and Gestalt process training in the early 2000s.

Gestalt therapy was an experiential therapy developed by Fritz Perls. Fritz Perls, Goodman Hefferline, and Paul Goodman. *Gestalt Therapy.* (New York: The Gestalt Journal Press, 1951).

155 *Good Sex Tool: Notice and Imagine:* I adapted this exercise from one of the processes used in the Radical Honesty trainings conducted by Brad Blanton.

156 *Good Sex Tool: Gestalt Hot Seat:* Brad Blanton created his own version of the classic Gestalt hot seat developed by Fritz Perls, which Brad uses in his workshops. I, in turn, created my own version of what I learned from Brad during Gestalt process trainings

with him. For information about hot seats and other Gestalt processes, see Thomas
A. Glass, "Gestalt Therapy," in *The Corsini Encyclopedia of Psychology* (Hoboken, NJ:
Wiley, 2010): 1–2.

158   *Good Sex Tool: Gestalt Life Story:* This is my version of a workshop exercise I learned
      from Brad Blanton during my Gestalt process trainings.
      Good Sex Tool: Journaling: There is extensive literature supporting the health benefits
      of journaling. James W. Pennebaker. *Writing to Heal: A Guided Journal for Recover-
      ing from Trauma & Emotional Upheaval* (Oakland, CA: New Harbinger Publications,
      2004); Keith J. Petrie et al. "Effect of Written Emotional Expression on Immune
      Function in Patients with Human Immunodeficiency Virus Infection: A Random-
      ized Trial," *Psychosomatic Medicine* 66, no. 2 (2004): 272–75; and Joan E. Broder-
      ick, Doerte U. Junghaenel, and Joseph E. Schwartz. "Written Emotional Expression
      Produces Health Benefits in Fibromyalgia Patients," *Psychosomatic Medicine* 67, no. 2
      (2005): 326–34.

8. Sex as a Tool for Transformation

162   *The Sex and Gender Continuum:* For an overview see chapter 7, "LUSTful Passions of
      the Mind," in Panksepp, *The Archaeology of Mind.*
      Going forward, for males, if development continues normally: The hormone DHT is re-
      sponsible for masculinizing the male genitals. S. M. Breedlove. "Sexual Differentia-
      tion of the Brain and Behavior," in J. B. Becker, S. M. Breedlove, & D. Crews (Eds.),
      Behavioral Endocrinology (Cambridge, MA: MIT Press, 1992).

163   *The brain, on the other hand, is a whole different story:* The brain is masculinized when
      testosterone is converted to estrogen by aromatase. P. Berta et al. "Genetic Evidence
      Equating SRY and Testis-Determining Factor," *Nature,* 348 (1990): 448–50.
      The question becomes: The developing female brain is not masculinized by estrogen
      prenatally because it is protected by alpha-fetoproteins that block that action of es-
      trogen on the chromosomally female brain. Bridget M. Nugent et al. "Brain Femini-
      zation Requires Active Repression of Masculinization Via DNA Methylation," *Nature
      Neuroscience* 18, no. 5 (2015): 690.

164   *Men and Women Are Indeed Different:* Organizing effects of hormones typically occur
      during prenatal development/shortly after birth — and tend to affect the structure of
      the body and brain, usually irreversibly. Activating effects of hormones, on the other
      hand, can happen at any time and vary as hormone levels shift; for example, some of
      the changes that happen at puberty. Garrett, *Brain & Behavior.*

165   *While it might be considered politically incorrect:* The "receptive fields" or places for tes-
      tosterone to have influence are plentiful in the male brain. Panksepp, *The Archaeology
      of Mind,* Kindle edition, 250–51.
      On the other hand, if all goes well during embryonic development: Estrogen and pro-

gesterone promote expansion of the oxytocin-receptive fields in the female brain. Panksepp, *The Archaeology of Mind,* Kindle edition, 256.

Another fascinating aspect of female sexuality is that women's interest in the erotic can wax and wane in response to cyclical changes in brain chemistry: A. J. Wilcox et al. "On the Frequency of Intercourse around Ovulation: Evidence for Biological Influences," *Human Reproduction* 19, no. 7 (2004): 1539–43.

Also, in women, arousal of the genitals (as measured by blood flow) doesn't translate into subjective sexual arousal or feeling turned on. Meredith L. Chivers and J. Michael Bailey. "A Sex Difference in Features that Elicit Genital Response," *Biological Psychology* 70, no. 2 (2005): 115–20.

166 *At first, in the early days, sexuality research by Masters and Johnson:* W. H. Masters and V. E. Johnson. *Human Sexual Response* (Boston, MA: Little, Brown, 1966); H. S. Kaplan. *Disorders of Sexual Desire and Other New Concepts and Techniques in Sex Therapy* (New York: Brunner/Hazel Publications, 1979); J. R. Berman and J. Bassuk. "Physiology and Pathophysiology of Female Sexual Function and Dysfunction," *World Journal of Urology* 20, no. 2 (2002): 111–18.

167 *Several sexologists, including Beverly Whipple and K. B. Brash-McGeer and Rosemary Basson:* Rosemary Basson. "Using a Different Model"; B. Whipple and K. B. Brash-McGreer. "Management of Female Sexual Dysfunction," in M. L. Sipski and C. J. Alexander (Eds.) *Sexual Function in People with Disability and Chronic Illness. A Health Professional's Guide* (Gaithersburg: Aspen Publishers; 1997): 509–34; K. Wylie and S. Mimoun. "Sexual Response Models in Women," *Maturitas* 63 no. 2: 112–15; Richard D. Hayes. "Circular and Linear Modeling of Female Sexual Desire and Arousal," *Journal of Sex Research* 48, no. 2–3 (2011): 130–41.

Spontaneous Versus Responsive Desire: Panksepp notes that males have gonads on the brain, whereas sexuality for females is far more complex and far less well understood. "It is almost as if boys had a bigger set of sex glands right within their brains, corresponding to the more obvious external gonads," Panksepp, *The Archaeology of Mind,* Kindle edition, 250–51.

170 *As mentioned earlier, what I've just described is the phenomenon called "new relationship energy," or NRE:* Semir Zeki. "The Neurobiology of Love," *FEBS Letters* 581, no. 14 (2007): 2575–79.

What's going on when we are revved up on NRE?: D. Marazziti and D. Canale. "Hormonal Changes When Falling in Love," *Psychoneuroendocrinology,* 29, no. 7 (2004), 931–36; Richard Delorme et al. "Platelet Serotonergic Predictors of Clinical Improvement in Obsessive Compulsive Disorder," *Journal of Clinical Psychopharmacology* 24, no. 1 (2004): 18–23.

Another finding is that levels of nerve growth factor, a neurotrophin: Enzo Emanuele et al. "Raised Plasma Nerve Growth Factor Levels Associated with Early-Stage Romantic Love," Psychoneuroendocrinology 31, no. 3 (2006): 288–94.

174 *What Is Your Erotic Fingerprint*: I call it "unique erotic fingerprints" rather than libido
     types, as did Sandra Pertot, since more than LUST is involved. It has lots to do with
     our bio/psycho/social fingerprints in addition to where we are in any moment on
     the desire curve and in terms of what is happening in our relationship. Sandra Pertot.
     *When Your Sex Drives Don't Match: Discover Your Libido Types to Create a Mutually
     Satisfying Sex Life* (Boston, MA: Da Capo Lifelong Books, 2007).

182 *Sometimes emotional imbalances within relationships or disconnects between two people
     can be addressed in reimagining gender roles*: The map of the four quadrants of Tan-
     tric masculine/feminine active/passive explored in this section was the product of
     personal communication I had with Dr. Rudy Ballantine in the late nineties. Rudy
     is a gifted physician and pioneered the integration of conventional and alternative
     approaches to healing. He was of the first American physicians to study Ayurveda in
     India. Rudolph Ballentine. *Radical Healing: Integrating the World's Great Therapeutic
     Traditions to Create a New Transformative Medicine* (New York: Three Rivers Press,
     1999); Rudolph Ballantine. *Kali Rising: Foundation Principles of Tantra for a Trans-
     forming Planet* (Ballentine, SC: Tantrikster Press, 2010).

186 *And reciprocally, by rebooting our sexual pleasure, we set in motion a cascade of beneficial
     neurochemicals*: Kringelbach, "Towards a functional neuroanatomy."

9. Good Sex Versus Great Sex: Embracing Your Sexual Potential

196 *Extraordinary lovers share qualities that have been explored in research spearheaded by the
     Canadian sexologist Peggy Kleinplatz*: Peggy J. Kleinplatz. "Learning from Extraordi-
     nary Lovers," *Journal of Homosexuality,* 50, no. 2–3 (2006), 325–48.

197 *In fact, according to Kleinplatz*: Peggy J. Kleinplatz. *New Directions in Sex Therapy: In-
     novations and Alternatives* (Abingdon, UK: Routledge, 2013). Even with additional
     clitoral stimulation, less than half of women (43 percent) report experiencing orgasm
     through intercourse 75 percent of the time. Debby Herbenick et al. "Women's Ex-
     periences with Genital Touching, Sexual Pleasure, and Orgasm: Results from a US
     Probability Sample of Women Ages 18 to 94," *Journal of Sex & Marital Therapy* 44, no.
     2 (2018): 201–12.

201 *Good Sex Tool: Touch Plus Imagery*: This exercise was inspired by the results of my
     study in which "just thinking" about genital stimulation activated sensory and reward
     brain regions similarly to that of pleasurable physical stimulation of the genitals and
     orgasm. Nan J. Wise. "Activation of Sensory Cortex."

203 *Good Sex Tool: Sensate Focus: Healthy Hedonism Version*: Masters and Johnson devel-
     oped the sensate focus exercises to help clients get out of spectatoring and into expe-
     riencing sensations of giving and receiving touch. They noticed that people who were
     comfortable being sexual had certain characteristics. They touched their partners for
     their own experience and focused on their sensations rather than trying to arouse

their partners. And lastly, they were effective in noticing when they would become distracted and were effective in harnessing their own attention and refocusing on the sensations of the experience.

The first phase of sensate focus excludes the genitals and breasts. The activities are gradually extended to be inclusive of breasts and genitals, and then mutual touching, and then eventually onto sexual intercourse as indicated. Masters. *Human Sexual Inadequacy*; Linda Weiner and Constance Avery-Clark. "Sensate Focus: Clarifying the Masters and Johnson's Model," *Sexual and Relationship Therapy* 29, no. 3 (2014): 307–19.

Index